Reconstructing Womanhood, Reconstructing Feminism

Reconstructing Womanhood, Reconstructing Feminism is the first British feminist anthology to examine concepts of womanhood and feminism within the context of 'race' and ethnicity. Challenging contemporary feminist theory, the book highlights the ways in which constructions of womanhood have traditionally excluded Black women's experience – and proposes a reconsideration of terms such as 'feminist'.

The research subjects and methods of many of the contributors have been shaped by the specifics of the Black British experience and context. Representing a variety of backgrounds including sociology, literary criticism, history and cultural theory, the collection makes new information accessible, adds fresh nuances to well-explored areas, reexamines old ideologies and uncovers previously concealed ones.

This volume brings together various perspectives about 'difference' and identity. It covers a diverse range of social and cultural issues including the position of Black women in the church, lesbian identity in fiction, contemporary African feminism, and British immigration law.

Delia Jarrett-Macauley is a writer, a researcher into Black women's history and feminist politics in Britain, and an arts management consultant.

Reconstructing Womanhood, Reconstructing Feminism

Writings on Black Women

Edited by Delia Jarrett-Macauley

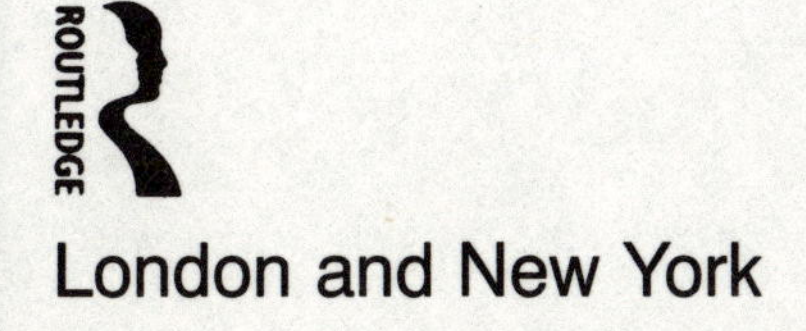

London and New York

First published 1996
by Routledge
11 New Fetter Lane, London EC4P 4EE

Simultaneously published in the USA and Canada
by Routledge
29 West 35th Street, New York, NY 10001

Phototypeset in Times by Intype, London
Printed and bound in Great Britain by
Clays Ltd, St Ives plc

British Library Cataloguing in Publication data
A catalogue record for this book is available from the British Library

Library of Congress Cataloguing in Publication Data
A catalogue record for this book has been requested

ISBN 0-415-11648-1 (hbk)
ISBN 0-415-11649-X (pbk)

For my mother,
Lily Macauley

Contents

Part II

Contributors

Ama Ata Aidoo was a lecturer at the University of Cape Coast, 1970–83, and Minister for Education (Ghana), 1982–83. Her numerous novels and anthologies have been widely published and translated, including *No Sweetness Here* (1970, Longman) and *Changes – A Love Story* (1991, The Women's Press). Ama is currently a full-time writer, living in Harare.

Valentina Alexander is completing a PhD on the response to oppression within the Black Led Churches in Britain at Warwick University. She has carried out freelance training in Black studies, Black women's literature, creative writing and Black theology and history, and has also coordinated and taught on Saturday schools and other Africentric child development programmes.

Helen (charles) is an activist and writer, giving lectures and facilitating workshops at a variety of organizations, groups and educational institutions. Her recent publications include chapters in S. Wilkinson and C. Kitzinger (eds) *Heterosexuality: Feminism and Psychology Reader* (1993, Sage) and in J. Bristow and A. Wilson *Activating Theory: Lesbian, Gay, Bisexual Politics.* The shape of her name reflects the origin of many Black family names in the nomenclature of European slave-owners.

Deborah Cheney is a lecturer in criminal law at the University of Kent. She is the author of *Into the Dark Tunnel – Foreign Prisoners in the British Prison System* (1993, Prison Reform Trust) and *The Foreign Prisoner Resource Pack* (Prison Reform Trust and HM Prison Service). Deborah is the Executive Committee member of the Association of Members of Boards of Visitors, and Editor of the journal *AMBoV Quarterly.*

Juliette Jarrett was educated at St Martin's School of Art and at the Institute of Education, London University. She is currently programme manager for Science and Technological courses at Lambeth College, South London.

Delia Jarrett-Macauley is a writer and has researched and taught Black women's history and feminist politics in Britain and the Caribbean. She was a lecturer in Women's Studies at the University of Kent from 1989–94. Since the 1980s she has worked in cultural management – on which she now lectures in Europe.

Annecka Marshall is completing a doctorate in sociology at the University of Warwick where she is also a part-time tutor. She has taught feminism and anti-racist courses for both the University of North London and for Birkbeck College, London University.

Felly Nkweto Simmonds is a senior lecturer in sociology at the University of Northumbria at Newcastle. Her recent publications include chapters in H. Hinds *et al.* (eds) *Working Out: New Directions for Women's Studies* (1992, Falmer Press) and in T. Lovell (ed.) *British Feminist Thought* (1990, Basil Blackwell).

Lola Young is Senior Lecturer in Media and Cultural Studies at Middlesex University and has written extensively on issues of 'race', gender and representation in films. Her book *Fear of the Dark: 'Race', Gender and Sexuality in the Cinema* was published by Routledge in late 1995.

Editor's introduction

There is a picture in my room,
It is a picture
Of a beautiful white lady
I used to think her sweet
But now I think
She lacks something.
I was so ugly
Because I am black
But now I am glad I am black
There is something about me
That has a dash in it
Especially when I put on
My bandanna.

(Marson, 'Black is fancy', 1937)

Of all the poems I know about Black women's ability to find beauty in themselves, in the face of negative stereotypes, this one is particularly important to me. Written long before the slogan, 'Black is Beautiful' became the vogue, it evokes a transforming moment in which the poet recognizes the need to abandon anything which would impede her sensitive development and fulfilment. More than half a century later, this poem affirmed my desire to encourage other Black women to put their dash into British scholarship. This book is, in part, the fruit of that desire. It is about the need to reject obsolete images and instead enjoy the enormous flexibility of self-definition.

The denial of freedom of self-expression which began with chattel slavery in the sixteenth century has taken many forms. African people, whether living on the continent or as part of the growing African Diaspora, have been recast in colonial and racist images as sexual, deviant, bestial, 'Other'. The stereotypes persisted, multiplied like lice, and found their way into every form of contemporary media. As the Trinidad-born activist Claudia Jones wrote in 1949:

> In the film, radio and press, the Negro woman is not pictured in her real role as breadwinner, mother and protector of the family, but as a traditional 'mammy' who puts the care of children and families of others above her own. This traditional stereotype of the Negro slave mother, which to this day appears in commercial advertisements, must be combatted and rejected as a device of the imperialist to perpetuate the white chauvinist ideology that Negro women are 'backward', 'inferior' and the 'natural slaves of others'.
>
> (quoted in Johnson 1984)

Black women in Britain today represent a permanent and talented part of the community, and yet Britain has responded to them in only the most grudging way. Still, for all the hype and the hyperbole which surrounds 'Black womanhood', we are still under-produced, under-explored, under-researched. We are a long way from the dynamic cultural and literary activities of African-Americans and in any event, our specific histories are quite different, as are the political practices and ideologies that have developed out of these.

But we have not been silent. From the early 1950s when significant numbers of West African and West Indian people arrived in Britain, we have learnt how to negotiate the island's selective welcome in both public and private spheres. This hands-on education has ranged from dealing with hostile neighbours, understanding the possible strains of ethnically mixed intimate relationships, to challenging the lack of accountability enjoyed by immigration officials, headteachers or doctors. The lesssons of the 1950s and 1960s sunk in deep, and we have long since graduated to new schools. Since the early 1980s there have been a number of published works by and about Black women in Britain. The majority of these are creative works, some of which are implicitly critical of Euro-American feminist theory.[1] A handful of non-fiction works published during the last decade have raised awareness of the position of Black women in this society; (Amos and Parmar 1984; Bryan *et al.* 1985; Mama 1984; Ngcobo 1988). Two of these deserve special mention. In 1984 the West African psychologist Amina Mama, in calling for more theoretical work on Black women in Britain, wrote that:

> a major objective of such work must be to develop appropriate conceptual tools and well-grounded theory. By this I mean grounded in the experiences and realities of the specific Black women concerned, and which incorporates the contingency of action on experience.
>
> (Mama 1984: 22)

This anthology has taken these words to heart.

Heart of the Race (Bryan *et al.* 1985), a Black female chorale, documented the forms and extent of sexual/racial discrimination in education, employment and the health service, as well as illuminating Black women's cultural work and political practice. On a theoretical level this work demonstrated that the different versions of the theory of capitalist patriarchy, which presupposed a unified female subject, did not adequately explain Black women's experience.

In spite of such writings and the increasing political activism of Black women's groups during the early 1980s, academic curricula, in line with much social policy and much feminist theory, failed to take account of our experiences or our words. Rarely has space been ceded to Black women's studies as an autonomous area in Britain because, it is generally claimed, no appropriate texts or experts existed. The problem is seen as one of invisibility.

The women's movement and the structures which have grown out of it are struggling with the politics of 'difference'. Today in the 1990s, any taken-for-granted notion of 'woman' is up for scrutiny and subject to change:

We are not all sisters under the same moon

and the moon is never the same two nights
running into different shapes choosing
to light up a certain crescent or to be
full and almost round or to slide into
a slither tilted backwards looking up to the stars.

Before this night is over and before
this new dawn rises we have to see
these particular changes speak to

our guarded uncertain before singing
Sisterhood is Powerful. Once we see
that light reflect our various colours;
when we feel complexity clear as an orange sun
moving into the morning maybe we can sit
here in the shade and talk
meeting each other's eyes with a sparkle
that is not afraid to see the lone bright poppy
nor afraid to question the dent
in the dream or the words missing
from the story.

When you see my tone
changes with the sun or ill health
when you realise
I am Not a Definition
perhaps we can move on.

For I am not only a strong woman
with a Scorpio rising I am
not about to dance with daffodils
everyday making putty out of my wishes
to shape my future needs. I have no
definite tomorrow only a longing that
I will write to pick out lights
that cast curious shadows in the dark.

And yes it would be easy to pat
the back of my confidence
smacking out my fears with assurance
saying strong women never hesitate:
looking inward into this particular
Black woman helps me look outward;
only by questioning the light
in my eyes can I refuse to be
dazzled by the lie in yours –
we are not all sisters
under the same moon.

(Kay, *A Dangerous Knowing* n.d.)

Most of the contributors to this collection are women living in Britain whose research subjects and methods are shaped by the specifics of the Black British experience and context. They draw on the recent writings of other Black women here: (Carby 1982; Grewal *et al.* 1988) and of African-American feminist theorists (Davis, 1981; Collins 1990 etc.; hooks 1981; Hull *et al.* 1982; Walker 1984) as well as diverse writers and theorists whose texts have formed Black consciousness worldwide, in particular Marcus Garvey, Frantz Fanon and Stuart Hall. However, their conceptual frameworks have emerged organically from their research rather than following the dictates of either fashion or alternative places.

The chapters in this book make new information accessible, add fresh nuances to well-explored areas, reexamine old ideologies and uncover previously concealed ones. All are informed, in a general sense, by a historical perspective and are concerned with reinterpreting the world in a way which includes Black women or specific groups of Black women. They vary in the extent to which some are highly specific, while others present more general theoretical analyses of the relation between ethnicity and gender.

The essays do not pretend at comprehensiveness, nor does this collection constitute a Black woman's charter. While the authors draw on biographical and autobiographical works, they are not arguing a personal case against discrimination. We are concerned with the difference between image and reality, policy and practice. Their words exist in the zones between exclusion/independence, imposition/resistance. They are concerned with the relationship between image and identity, representation and power, politics and culture.

The collection has grown out of my teaching courses on the MA in Women's Studies at the University of Kent from 1989 to 1994. The course – 'Historical and Contemporary Issues of Black Women in Britain' – was an inter-disciplinary exploration balanced towards history from chattel slavery in the British West Indies to present-day life in Britain. It employed a patchwork of texts ranging from W. E. B. Dubois' early twentieth-century classic, *The Souls of Black Folk* (1969) to Alice Walker's *In Search of Our Mother's Gardens* (1984); 'white'[2] feminist analyses such as Lynne Segal's *Is the Future Female?* (1987) and works generally unheralded in England such as *Jamaica Woman: An Anthology of Poems* (1980). The course – my introduction to university teaching – was both a serious academic undertaking and a very good game.

Some of the fun arose from the effort of replacing ourselves –

Black women in Britain and 'white' women studying Black British women for the first time – in texts which had not necessarily seen us coming. The success of the enterprise depended to a significant degree on our imaginative reconstructing of ideas; for example, how to insert a discussion around the politics of difference in women's creativity without denying the individuality of the artist. Or, how to 'hear' the voices of African-Caribbean slave women against the cacophony of those who abused, oppressed and exploited them. After a two-year run, I altered and renamed the course. It became Reconstructing Womanhood, Reconstructing Feminism, in recognition of the fact that identity and revisioning were now sitting jointly at its fulcrum – with history on one side.

In my complementary roles of writer/editor, teacher, I had two distinct, but related, aims. The first was to research Black women's lives in contemporary and historical fields and to increase the body of knowledge of that lived experience. The second was to look at the construction of images of the Black woman, whose status as 'Other' in literature, film and art has supported a system of domination and subordination in Euro-American thought and life. Accordingly, this anthology, which falls into two parts, reflects those interests.

NOTES

1 See for example the novels of Joan Riley, Vernella Fuller and Buchi Emecheta.
2 As 'whiteness' is generally not seen in terms of recognized ethnicity, and has not yet been widely researched, it is appropriate to highlight it as such. See Richard Dyer (1988) 'White', *Screen* 29(4): 44–64.

BIBLIOGRAPHY

Amos, V. and Parmar, P. (1984) 'Challenging imperial feminism' *Feminist Review* 17: 3–19.
Bryan, B., Dadzie, S. and Scafe, S. (1985) *Heart of the Race*, London: Virago.
Carby, H. (1982) 'White woman listen! Black feminism and the boundaries of sisterhood' in Centre for Contemporary Cultural Studies (ed.) *The Empire Strikes Back. Race and Racism in '70s Britain*, London: Hutchinson pp. 212–35.
Collins, P. H. (1990) *Black Feminist Thought*, London: HarperCollins.
Davis, A. (1981) *Women Race and Class*, London: Women's Press.

Dubois, W. E. B. (1969) *The Souls of Black Folk*, New York: NAL Penguin.
Dyer, R. (1988) 'White', *Screen* 29, 4: 44–64.
Grewal, S. (ed.) (1988) *Charting the Journey: Writings by Black and Third World Women*, Inland Womensource.
hooks, b. (1981) *Ain't I a Woman. Black Women and Feminism*, London: Pluto Press.
Hull, G., Scott, P. B. and Smith, B. (eds) (1982) *All the Women are White, All the Blacks are Men, But Some of Us are Brave*, New York: The Feminist Press.
Johnson, B. (1984) *'I think of My Mother': the Life of Claudia Jones*, London: Karia Press.
Kay, J. (n.d.) *A Dangerous Knowing. Four Black Women Poets*, London: Sheba Feminist Publishers.
Mama, A. (1984) 'Black women, the economic crisis and the British state' *Feminist Review* 17: 21–35.
Marson, U. (1937) 'Black is fancy' in *The Moth and the Star*, Kingston, Jamaica.
Mordecai, P. and Morris, M. (eds) (1980) *Jamaica Woman: An Anthology of Poems*, London and Kingston: Heinemann.
Ngcobo, L. (ed.) (1988) *Let It Be Told. Black Women Writers in Britain*, London: Virago.
Segal, L. (1987) *Is the Future Female?*, London: Virago.
Walker, A. (1984) *In Search of Our Mother's Gardens: Feminist Prose*, London: Women's Press.

Acknowledgements

Special thanks are due to Lyn Innes and Tina Papoulias for their welcome advice on some of the essays, and to Louisa John-Baptiste at Women's Training Link for invaluable administrative assistance and support.

I am grateful to Heather Gibson at Routledge for her encouragement and to Fiona Bailey and Christina Tebbit for their kindness and diligence.

Many teachers and family members have helped me over the years. Not least, I thank my friends for their love and support and for having faith in me. Some to whom I owe more than a nod of gratitude are Beverley Duguid, Susan Pennybacker, Nigel Pollitt, Beverley Randall, Juliette Verhoeven, Sheila Rowbotham and Jacqueline Young.

Part I

Introduction

These five essays are all grounded in the experiences of particular women – be they individual activists and writers or representatives of a wider contingent. But this is not a catalogue of personal life stories, nor a rhetorical burst on sexism and racism. The authors in this section use biography and autobiography, oral testimonies and interview material as a means of providing a panoramic description of the 'realities' of Black women's lives within the theoretical frameworks constructed through their research. In the main, they are concerned with external barriers to Black women's equality in Britain. Social and political structures which undermine Black women's lives – in education, employment and social services – are rarely subject to detailed scrutiny. Without such analysis the development of Black British feminist thought, and related feminist activism, is inevitably hindered.

Explicitly or implicitly, these pieces refer to the historical continuum which began with chattel slavery, led to colonialism and finally to the migration of African and African-Caribbean peoples to Britain after the Second World War. Indeed, many of the contemporary experiences of Black British women are explained by that specific history. For example, African-Caribbean women are the most economically active group of women in this society and yet they have very low economic status: these linked precedents date back to the period of slavery itself. However, although this historical continuum must be constantly borne in mind, the task of unwrapping our knowledge of Black women's lives is not the province of historians alone. Black feminism provides a method of working which enables these writers to come up with new answers to old questions and even new subjects for enquiry, and to make the experiences of Black women distinct from those of their 'white' female and/or Black male counterparts. From their various academic disciplines – art, literature, history, law and sociology, they imply that many textbooks need to be reviewed from a standpoint which is sensitive to the situation of Black women as a social group.

The subject-matter covered here is, of course, diverse. It ranges from considering religious participation within both 'white'-led and Black-led churches, to discussing the ideologies that support racist/sexist discrimination within the immigration service. There is an analysis of how 'external' images of Black womanhood corrupt personal relationships and how anxieties about Black female sexuality feed into those relationships. In addition, two essays approach questions of identity by exploring how effacement, exclusion and denial have shaped Black women's lives both historically and today.

Chapter 1

From sexual denigration to self-respect: resisting images of Black female sexuality

Annecka Marshall

The song *Respect* makes me think about the myriad of images that have been used both by 'white' people and Black men not only to deny us respect but to dominate us (Franklin 1967). Portraying Black women as sexually denigrated has been central to the ideological justification for systems of racism, sexism, heterosexism and class oppression. The historical development of representations of Black women as animalistic, diseased and licentious has contributed to our subordination in contemporary Britain. In this chapter I discuss the significance of the depiction of Black women as dirty, incapable of sexual morality and unable to control our lust. In particular I consider Black women's own perceptions of being stereotyped as sensuous, bestial, good in bed, loose, promiscuous, breeders and prone to prostitution. The objectification of Black women as creatures of sex not only influences our identity and relationships but, I argue, is also used by 'white' people and Black men to legitimize our sexual and social exploitation. I conclude by discussing the creation of positive self-definitions as a powerful challenge to the ways in which derogatory myths have been oppressive for Black women. We resist negative images by asserting our right to define our identities and to control our sexuality.

SENSUOUS SLAVERY

Since slavery, images of Black women as hypersexual have been used to justify our sexual exploitation and, as such, have contributed to our inferior socioeconomic and political position in Britain. During slavery the belief that Africans were sub-human savages with uncontrollable sexual capacities was used to legitimate the exploitation of their labour. The image of the sexually aggressive woman has from the sixteenth century contributed to the institutionalization of efforts to control us. As Black women were relegated to the category of sensuous slaves this provided a forceful legitimation for their sexual abuse by 'white' men. I will later demonstrate that economic exploitation was evident in the ways in which Black women's sexuality was linked to their fertility – since Black women were seen as possessing excessive sexual appetites, increased fertility was expected. In the modern era these images have been transformed to have new meanings and functions, which though obviously not as insidious as during the days of enslavement, nevertheless have similar effects.

The sexual overtones that have become embedded in ideas about racial difference are eloquently analysed by Winthrop Jordan. He argues that when English voyagers initially explored West Africa in 1550 they regarded the Africans they encountered as radically apart from and different to themselves. Jordan explains that by the middle of the sixteenth century English people believed that Africans were different in terms of their skin colour and associated this with an unChristian religion as well as libidinousness. I intend to assess the development of such stereotypes, and the ways in which it was taken for granted that Africans were carefree, lazy and lustful cannibals. Even before African slaves were brought to England from the 1570s onwards, the perception of their sexual degeneration was deep within the English psyche. Partly these impressions were for English people a means to interrogate themselves by means of comparison (Jordan 1982).

Jordan argues that from the middle of the sixteenth century four factors structured the English view of the African as a slave. First, the African's skin colour was seen in a negative way. In England the concept of Blackness was equated with sin and flirtatiousness. Indeed Blackness was the antithesis of 'whiteness'. 'whiteness' symbolized purity, virginity, virtue, beauty, beneficence and God. In contrast Blackness connoted filthiness, sin, baseness, ugliness, evil and the devil. Second, the African was considered to be a heathen and uncivilized. As such, extensive English involvement in the slave trade during the seventeenth century was rationalized as being a civilizing mission. Third, the African was viewed as a savage beast. In particular the English associated

Africans with apes – a central idea to which I will return as it is quite pertinent to present-day imagery. This association is clearly shown by the notion of sexual unions between Africans and apes:

> The sexual association of apes with Negroes had an inner logic which kept it alive: sexual union seemed to prove a certain affinity without going so far as to indicate actual identity which was what Englishmen really thought was the case. By forging a sexual link between Negroes and apes, furthermore, Englishmen were able to give vent to their feeling that Negroes were a lewd, lascivious, and wanton people.
>
> (Jordan 1982: 52–3)

Lastly, the African was perceived as being sexually potent. Linking Africans with animality was fraught with sexual connotations. In fact sexual indulgence was seen as a sign of inferiority and social backwardness. This is important because English people used Africans as social mirrors, and projected characteristics onto them which they had originally discovered in themselves. Jordan argues that as a result of the English reaction to their initial contacts with Africans – equating Blackness with aggressive sexuality and evil – it was maintained that strict discipline and moral control was necessary (ibid.). Moreover, the myth of the super-sexual Black is especially interesting in view of English society's repressed attitude towards sexuality. The image of Black sexual deviancy was reinforced by and confirmed Western bourgeois standards for the control of sexual passions. Black women were differentiated from 'white' women in a sexual sense; the former were defined as sexually immoral and promiscuous, whereas the latter were elevated as chaste and passionless. Stereotypes of heightened sexuality were, as Barbara Bush explains in her brilliant analysis, used to justify the sexual abuse of Black women by 'white' men. 'White' men transferred the blame for their sexual improprieties onto the evil charms of Black women and so exonerated themselves:

> With the rise of Christianity, sexuality came to be associated with the devil and the colour black to symbolise all the evil and sinful elements in life. As women in Europe were traditionally regarded as instigators of evil-doing, Blackness was also associated with femininity; hence the link between the delights of a forbidden sexuality would have easily (and possibly almost

unconsciously) been made by European men during their initial contacts with African societies.

(Bush 1990: 14)

Black sexuality was associated with earthiness, impurity, indecency and corruption and as such represented the antithesis of the ideal of English sexual mores. As I have previously mentioned Black people were compared to, and it was believed mated with, animals. Thomas Jefferson maintained that the combination of animal intelligence and human form in the Black 'race' was the result of sexual intercourse between the orangutan and the Black female (Fryer 1988). Similarly the French naturalist Buffoon claimed that the primitive, lascivious and ape-like sexual appetites of Blacks encouraged Black women to copulate with apes (ibid.).

In the same way as these images were used to justify slavery, from the late eighteenth century theories of biological determinism legitimated inequalities of status, power and wealth (ibid.). Pseudo-scientific arguments that identify and set apart Black people as not only physically distinct in terms of 'race' but also in terms of sexuality have supported ideologies of Black inferiority and the preservation of 'white' bourgeois domination. During the nineteenth century it was claimed that the inherent abnormality and pathology of Black female genitalia signified that Blacks were a separate and lower race (Gilman 1985).

Thereby the genitalia of the Black woman indicated that she was diseased, bestial and unapproachable. The contradictory sexualized figure of Blacks was linked to genitalia that were defined as complete yet damaged, diseased yet attractive, poisoning yet potent (ibid.). Consequently Black female genitalia represented sexual pathology, corruption and death. Sander Gilman asserts that the fear and fascination of Black difference ensured that Black women were despised, forbidden yet sexually exploited (ibid.). Hence sexual contact with Black women were regarded as debasing but also exciting, and it follows that Black women have been described as and ascribed the role of prostitutes. The female slave was considered to be governed almost entirely by her libido. Her sexual attributes were often sensationally exaggerated as offering the delights of illicit sex. Enslaved Black women were sexually objectified as loose, lewd and wanton. The argument that Black women were lascivious and immoral was used to rationalize their sexual abuse by 'white' masters and overseers. According to Alice Walker:

> For centuries the black woman has served as the primary pornographic 'outlet' for white men in Europe and America. We need only think of the black women used as breeders, raped for the pleasure and profit of their owners. We need only think of the license the 'master' of the slave women enjoyed. But, most telling of all, we need only study the old slave societies of the South to note the sadistic treatment – at the hands of white 'gentlemen' – of 'beautiful young quadroons and octoroons' who became increasingly (and were deliberately bred to become) indistinguishable from white women, and were the most highly prized as slave mistresses because of this.
>
> (Walker 1981: 42)

Under enslavement the endeavours of slave-owners to increase the fertility of Black women in order to maximize profits entailed the systematic control of the sexuality of female slaves. The actual breeding of slave women served to label them as animalistic as well as to maintain their treatment as less than human, since only animals can be bred against their will. Within the breeding system the exploitation of Black female reproductive labour was justified by sexually denigrating Black women. Thus the portrayal of Black women as libidinous was used to gratify the sexual and economic needs of 'white' male slave-owners and managers (Collins 1990). Patricia Hill Collins validates this point in her erudite analysis of the economic advantages that accrued to the image of the Black woman as a breeder. Collins asserts that:

> controlling Black women's reproduction was essential to the creation and perpetuation of capitalist class relations. Slavery benefitted certain segments of the population by economically exploiting others. . . . Under such a system in which the control of property is fundamental, enslaved African women were valuable commodities. Slaveowners controlled Black women's labour and commodified Black women's bodies as units of capital. Moreover, as mothers, Black women's fertility produced the children who increased their owners' property and labour force.
>
> (Collins 1990: 51)

The sexual violation of Black women by 'white' men symbolized a wider system of 'white' male domination. As Angela Davis argues, sexual exploitation under slavery was an institutionalized method of terrorism that aimed to demoralize and dehumanize slave women as well as slave men (Davis 1982).

Since slavery, stereotyping Black women as sexually denigrated has been instrumental to our subordination. The relegation of Black women to the status of sexual animals has reaffirmed Western ideals of sexual purity, morality and social order. Sander Gilman stresses that Black people represented the converse of European sexual mores and beauty. Black women were perceived as more primitive and therefore more sexually intense. Their essence was defined in terms of their genitalia. Western notions of 'race', sexuality and pathology are fascinating because they constitute a means by which the European male copes with his anxieties concerning his control over the world. Gilman emphasizes that a secure definition of self is maintained by projecting the loss of sexual control onto Blacks, who symbolize dirt, decay and unbridled sexuality:

> the ' "white" man's burden', his sexuality and its control, is displaced into the need to control the sexuality of the Other, the Other as sexualized female.
>
> (Gilman 1985: 107)

Relatedly, Homi Bhabha argues that the association of Blackness with savagery, cannibalism, anarchy and lust not only represents the transference of 'white' ambivalence but the vindication of the oppression of Black people (Bhabha 1983).

The definition of self is very important in my analysis. I will go on to show how a positive definition of self is essential for Black women to challenge stereotypes. This brief history of the construction of images of Black female sexuality demonstrates that images of Black women as the 'Others' within British society have constituted a form of social control. The depiction of Black women as supersexual beings has contributed to the definition of 'whites' as sexually restrained. The development and maintenance of images of Black female sexuality has been a primarily 'white' male and, to a lesser extent, 'white' female and Black male means of exerting authority over us. Since 'white' culture and Black patriarchy gained in strength and identity by defining Black female sexuality as inferior, these images still have currency. My concern about the pervasive impact of these images upon Black women's lives has motivated my present research. Although people are increasingly aware of the existence of such stereotypes, their effects and the actual opinions of Black women are less well known. Accordingly the rest of this chapter considers Black women's experiences of the construction of racist sexual images.

CONTEMPORARY IMAGES OF BLACK FEMALE SEXUALITY

Images of Black female sexuality that originated in the sixteenth century have, in various forms, continued to the present day. Whilst I focus in this section on Britain in the 1990s, I want to stress that since enslavement in Africa and the Diaspora, images of Black female sexuality have continued to hold the material interests of the 'white' male elite in many ways. Although these images differ in terms of historical and cultural specifics, their impact is similar in that they have structured a subordinate reality for Black women. The fact that this historical process has been largely hidden has inevitably helped to increase the pervasiveness of images and ideas about Black female sexuality. These images have become a central part of racist ideologies and practices. Before I embarked upon my research I was aware that as a Black woman I was seen by Black men and by 'white' people as a sexual fiend. As I was unaware of the historical legacy and because these views were presented as 'common sense', I found it difficult to resist them. Reading the literature and discussing these images with other Black women during the course of my research has helped me to understand their material significance. The incorporation of such notions into 'the British way of life' has effectively served to rationalize our oppression. The prevalent images of the Black female define her as sensuous and animalistic, as a prostitute, breeder or Sapphire.

Sensuous

When I interviewed 21 Black women about the extent to which the historical construction of Black sexuality is still relevant, they explained that they were dominantly objectified and associated with sensuousness. The stereotype of the sensuous Black female is omnipresent. Tracy Ross is a 32-year-old research worker who believes that this image also incorporates the idea that Black women are mystical, fiery and licentious. Tracy thinks that 'white' men fantasize about Black women being over-sexed but regard us to be a taboo:

> 'I think that many of the sexual images are sensual images. Black women are seen as sensually appealing. Often there's this dark mystical woman. Often Black women's figures, their shapes, are very different to "white" women and so they're much more ample both above and below. I think that's seen as very sensual. I often think it's seen as off limits. It's seen as if it's hot; it's too hot to handle.'

Whilst it is generally argued that 'white' men promote an image of Black women as sensuous there is disagreement about the degree to which this influences the likelihood of inter-racial relationships. Tracy maintains that due to this stereotype 'white' men tend to be scared of approaching Black women, whereas Yvonne Stewart, a 39-year-old legal secretary, argues to the contrary. Yvonne considers the contradiction between a portrayal of Black women that stresses our hypersexuality, and so does not allow for differences that exist among us, and her contention that Black women *are* in fact sexy;

> 'They look better. Black women do look sexy. That's all there is to it really. They are very sexy women. They have this thing, don't they? And yes, I suppose "white" men do find them sexy. I'll tell you a "white" man said to me "you're all woman". He had the hots for me. He drove me crazy. We have this image, I suppose, of being sexy and we are. It's really hard for me to say on a whole. I'm just like speaking on a personal level because I really don't know. Sometimes I can't understand Black women themselves myself.'

How powerful is the image of Black women's sex appeal? The internalization of racist stereotypes will be addressed in the next section. At present I want to demonstrate that the legacy of these stereotypes has profound implications for analyses of racism in Britain. As Frantz Fanon highlights in his psychoanalytic interpretation of the fact of Blackness: 'if one wants to understand the racial situation psychoanalytically . . . as it is experienced by individual consciousness, considerable importance must be given to sexual phenomena.' (1970: 160)

For Black women being seen as sensuous is linked to broader negative connotations. According to Joel Kovel the sexualized nature of racist psychology is intimately connected with issues of power, dominance and status. The sexual symbolism and fantasies underlying racism is evident in 'white' people's perception of Black people as 'warm, dirty, sloppy, feckless, lazy, improvident and irrational, all those traits that are associated with Blackness, odour, and sensuality (Kovel 1970: 195).

Animalistic

Since the eighteenth century pseudo-scientific racism has connected Black sexuality with animal imagery. Today Black women are battling against this notion in order to gain recognition of our common humanity. Hence Sally B., a 32-year-old housing officer, complains that the portrayal of Black women as animalistic and lustful is seen as justifying our abuse:

> 'It is "white" men who see the Black woman as an unsatisfied mamma just to be used sexually . . . Black women are seen as sexual animals. For example, in the media they are beasts. The Black woman is an unsatiated mamma who can satisfy you. You are just to be used any way and not to be seen as a person. As a human being you are used and thrown away like rubbish.'

Relatedly the contention that Black women are only good in bed has meant that we are subsumed to a sexual role that denies us credence elsewhere. There are diverse ways of coping with this.

Yvonne Stewart tries to ignore the myth that Black women are better in bed than 'white' women. Others analyse the images. The link between this stereotype and that of Black women's animal-like sexuality is explored by Sian Lacy, a 24-year-old trainee solicitor. She suggests that within the notion of an animal-like sexuality is the belief that Black women are sexually wild, strong and passionate. Moreover, the Black woman is regarded as being 'a woman who can fuck'. Sian rejects the icon of the oversexed Black woman. She thinks that the view that Black women are good at sex and give as good as we get sexually, dehumanizes us to a sort of working animal. As such the subjugation of Black women entails the historical legacy of being a workhorse under the yoke. Sian believes:

> 'I suppose we're seen as just there to do whatever is necessary. So if you meet somebody's services sexually you will fulfil that role as well.'

Loose

Interlinked with ideas about Black female sexual proclivity is the concept of being easily available. Melisa Jones, a 26-year-old office supervisor, maintains that 'white' men are fascinated by the way that Black women look. She thinks that because Black women have a different skin colour from 'whites' it is also held to be an indication that Black women possess different sexual attributes. This supports Sander L. Gilman's analysis of the correlation between 'race', sexuality and pathology. Gilman asserts that:

> Sexual anatomy is so important a part of self-image that 'sexually different' is tantamount to 'pathological' – the other is 'impaired', 'sick', 'diseased'. Similarly, physiognomy or skin colour that is perceived as different is immediately associated with 'pathology' and 'sexuality'.
>
> (1985: 25)

Therefore, by virtue of our phenotypical characteristics, Black women are seen as inherently sexual as well as sick. Consequently the stereotype of Black women being sexually adventurous, laid back and letting ourselves go is interpreted as a sign of pathology. Melisa discusses the prevalence of the view that Black women 'enjoy themselves, roll about more, are more lively, willing and able'. According to Melisa, 'white' men are curious about Black women because:

> 'coloured girls are supposed to be more sexually aware. They let themselves go more. This is why I think that some "white" guys go out with Black girls. Now they all want to have a go. They want to know if it's really true. People want to know what the fascination is. I think they're fascinated by the hype that we've got. . . . It starts off with the fascination and then it gets hyped up. And then the fascination just escalates and it stays there.'

Thus as Gilman argues, the concept of racial difference is ingrained with sexual meanings. Within a racist society the conjunction of 'race' and sexuality often leads to 'white' people having many fantasies about Blacks (ibid.). This is shown by the general assertion that in British society and the mass media there are myths about promiscuous Black women. Whilst it is assented that in the main 'white' men propagate these myths there is some dispute about the extent to which 'white' women and Black men do also. Roseanne Park, a 22-year-old student, argues that the image of promiscuity is so pervasive that often Black men also believe it. This not only allows Black men to resist being defined in the same category as Black women, but also enables them to maintain patriarchal power. Roseanne argues that:

> 'It is an image because it's untrue. It's a racist way of keeping Black women down. It has worked because the Black man uses the view that she is promiscuous; because it ties in with the whole idea of her being independent and head of the household. The Black man is almost led by the hand to believe this because he has already been told that she wears the trousers. He doesn't challenge that so he isn't going to challenge that she's a slut in bed. He just goes along with it because it makes his life easier. It gives him an explanation as to why he's not doing so well.'

Prostitute

The obvious conclusion to the theory that Black women are promiscuous is that we are prone to prostitution. Assessing the manner in which Black women are pathologized sexually Lola Young explains how we are:

> constructed through a white male fantasy which sees female genitalia as evidence of an anomalous sexuality and Black female sexuality as a sexual and social threat to be subjected to control. The Black woman is not only the object of sexual perversity, she is also its source. Alongside that, the belief that female prostitution is somehow a natural consequence of excessive female sexuality still has currency.
>
> (Young 1990: 195)

For Black women the caricature of the whore is not just

incidental but rather a constant hazard. This image permeates various institutions including the mass media, the welfare state and occupational settings (see Simmonds 1988). Fosuwa Andoh, a 31-year-old artist, discusses the 'mammy and whore' dichotomy:

> 'I think that on TV Black women are asexual or they go to the other extreme and they are prostitutes. . . . Those are the two extremes where they have no sexuality or they have too much.'

Breeder

In addition, the connection between the mammy and whore imagery is evident in the myth that Black women are good breeders. The portrayal of Black women as more sexually active than 'white' women as well as being bestial was used to legitimate the breeding system during slavery and it can be argued that it still exists today (Davis 1985). The legacy of this myth is demonstrated by the conviction that Black women in contemporary Britain are only fit for breeding. The stereotype of the strong Black female who is capable of having many children is not only regarded as pervasive among 'white' people; it is also claimed that some Black men believe this image and that this affects their treatment of Black women. Accordingly Beverley Marsden, a 47-year-old nurse, states that:

> 'Men just see us here as breeding animals. I don't think they see us as women who have a right to say what we want.'

Moreover, it is argued that the image of Black women as breeders constitutes an institutionalized tool to disempower us. Zora Day, a 29-year-old temp, condemns the widespread assertion that Black women can merely produce children. Zora's awareness that the image of the breeder influences Black women's access to benefits is also examined by Bryan *et al.* (1985). Zora argues that within social policies stereotype exists of women who migrate to Britain and are then too lazy to work. It is claimed that instead of contributing to the British economy we have too many children and are social scroungers. As a result Black women are blamed for the destruction of our own families as well as the welfare state. However, Bryan *et al.* criticize the image of Black women as parasites:

> We are described by the media as 'scroungers' and depicted as having a child-like dependence upon a benevolent caring (white) society. Social workers are seen as the twentieth century missionaries who come into our communities to challenge ignorance and poverty. This image does not, however, expose the extent to which social and economic factors outside our control have forced us into this cycle of dependency on the State; nor does it convey the true nature of our contribution to this society. Black women's labour has propped up this country, not only over the past four decades but for centuries. Far from draining its resources, we have been the producers of its wealth.
>
> (1985: 111)

The contradictions in images of Black womanhood are important. There is not one consistent image or meaning. Rather, images have changed with different historical contexts to maintain power hierarchies. During slavery the image of the breeder was used to rationalize the sexual exploitation of Black women in order to maximize profits. While in contemporary Britain, that same image is used to implement social sanctions to reduce our fertility, negating the requirements of the economic system. Both instances demonstrate that we can only comprehend attempts to control Black female sexuality and fertility when we acknowledge the requirements of a given hegemony.

Sapphire

Dominant ideas about Black womanhood are presented as a denial of 'normal' gender relations. In terms of rejecting the prescribed sexual scenario of submissive female and dominant male the Black woman is a threat to masculinity. This is evident in the Sapphire stereotype, which as bell hooks explains, shows Black women as assertive, tough and evil:

> As Sapphires, black women were depicted as evil, treacherous, bitchy, stubborn, and hateful, in short all that the mammy figure was not. The Sapphire image had at its base one of the oldest negative stereotypes of woman – the image of the female as inherently evil. Christian mythology depicted woman as the source of sin and evil; racist-sexist mythology simply designated black women the epitome of female evil and

> sinfulness. White men could justify their dehumanization and sexual exploitation of black women by arguing that they possessed inherent evil demonic qualities. Black men could claim that they could not get along with black women because they were so evil. And white women could use the image of the evil sinful black woman to emphasize their own innocence and purity. Like the biblical figure Eve, black women became the scapegoats for misogynist men and racist women who needed to see some group of women as the embodiment of female evil.
>
> (1982: 85)

By virtue of potentially challenging the sexual status quo Black women are defined as sinful, powerful and dangerous. Thus, Black women are stigmatized as being strong and predatory sexual temptresses. Furthermore, we are considered to have an innate ability to mesmerize and bewitch men. The pervasiveness of the Sapphire ideology and the interdependence of racialized sexual images is indicated by Roseanne Park:

> 'The myths are promoted basically by "white" people, particularly the "white" male in his quest to dominate Black people. Myths such as the Sapphire; the promiscuous Black woman. There's the idea that the Black woman can sleep around. It all goes back to a loose woman concept. That myth is created by the "white" man to maintain the power hierarchy.'

I want to emphasize that for Black women who are pathologized as sexually perverse and deviant such myths need to be understood within the socioeconomic and political context of our position in Britain. Since the subjugation of Black women is integral to the maintenance of present inequalities, racist stereotypes about Black women's sexuality should be seen as part of our subordination in British society. It is extremely difficult for Black women to move beyond these images because they are ingrained in popular consciousness. As such, our opportunities in areas like education, employment and housing are circumscribed.

Pressures against Black women getting out of this racialized and sexist ghetto are largely due to the latent peril that the possibility presents to 'whites'. Frantz Fanon explains 'white' people's fantasies about Blacks and how they are characterized by sexual anxiety and disgust.

Fanon examines 'whites' ' phobic reaction to Blacks – feelings of fear, revulsion and loathing. Racial conflict is due to 'white' people's insecurity about their own sexuality combined with a compulsion to control the sexuality of Black people. For 'whites' the uncontrollability of Black sexuality is further interpreted as a threat to systems of 'white' domination (Fanon 1970).

Lola Young argues that the anxiety that 'white' people have about their own sexual passions are projected onto Black people. Young believes that, for 'white' people, anxiety is due to a perception of a loss of control over their own sexual desires. Yet this anxiety is repressed by defining a secure image of 'white' people as in control of their sexual needs and constructing the inverse of this in Black people:

> For whites to see themselves as rational, ordered and civilised people, they have to construct a notion of irrationality, disorder and uncivilised behaviour which is then imposed on the object of their stimulus to anxiety. Elements of the culture which are repressed re-emerge in the despised culture. So that where whites may have fantasies about total sexual abandonment whilst living under a yoke of sexual repression, that fantasy is projected onto Blacks.
>
> (Young 1990: 193)

Therefore Young maintains that a crisis in 'white' sexual identity leads to a transference of anger, frustration and loss of control onto Blacks. Subsequently Blacks are seen as symbolic of nature, dirt and decay. Hence Black people are viewed as instinctual, diseased and tainted. By associating Blackness with alienation and chaos, Young asserts, 'white' people attempt to cope with their own desire and pain. Thereby Blacks, since we are seen as different and in opposition to 'whites', are identified as the source of disorder, corruption and violence (ibid.).

The contradictions between the idealized and the actual self; the former being the prevalent image of 'white' sexuality and the latter projected onto Black people, is extremely difficult to comprehend. One way of dealing with this dilemma is to split the self into good and bad. Illustrating this issue Sander Gilman asserts that:

> The 'bad' self, with its repressed sadistic impulses, becomes the 'bad' other; the 'good' self/object, with its infallible correctness,

> becomes the antithesis to the flawed image of the self, the self out of control. The 'bad' other becomes the negative stereotype; the 'good' other becomes the positive stereotype. The former is what we fear to become: the latter that which we cannot achieve.
>
> (1985: 20)

Common-sense ideas about Black women being 'sensuous', 'animalistic', 'good in bed', 'loose', 'promiscuous', 'prostitutes', 'breeders' and 'Sapphires' may be used by 'white' people to justify denying Black women equal access to social and economic resources as well as political rights. If it is admitted that these images are false then the nature of 'white' sexuality will also have to be reassessed. Consequently the ascription of negative characteristics is developed by the mass media so that Black women are defined as inferior. Thus myths about Black women's sexuality give rise to fascination, fear and resentment among many 'white' people. As such Black women's sexuality and the connection that is automatically made to a high rate of fertility is a source of racial antagonism and hostility. Since it is believed that Black female sexuality and fertility represent a threat to 'the British way of life' attempts are made to regulate it. The perceived damage that Black women's sexuality may do to the social order is controlled by reinforcing racist ideologies and the 'white' power to which they give rise.

These images contribute to Black women's sense of self in complex ways. Like all racist stereotyping more is known about the process of defining than the effects upon those who are defined. So although views about the social construction of Black female sexuality are beginning to be discussed, it is pertinent to consider how this is related to Black women's identification. Having established that in present-day Britain the circumstances of Black women cannot be separated from how we are portrayed in sexual terms, I will now contemplate the impact upon Black women's self-definitions. The point of this endeavour is not just to assess identity in itself but rather to highlight that autonomous Black female identification can be used to fight against the stereotypes.

IDENTITY AS EMPOWERMENT

How are our identities influenced by racialized sexual imagery? For me, consciousness of the attempts of 'white' people and Black men to categorize my sexuality as not only intrinsically different but also as deviant necessarily entails a wider strategy to challenge this. Through my own self-definition of my sexuality, which I must admit is often contradictory, I strive to regain the power that others have tried to deny me. Researching this issue is more than a vindication of Black femininity. By analysing these images and their impact on Black women I stress the need for attacking them on multiple levels. Personally in our perceptions of ourselves and within our relationships it is vital that Black women confront such myths. I strive to explore this potential through my academic work since I believe that increasing a general awareness of the prevalence of these images is crucial. The site of my resistance against these stereotypes is my experience as a PhD student and as a lecturer. When I do research, write or lecture I endeavour to encourage the 'audience' to debunk racist, sexist, homophobic and elitist ideologies and practices. Incarcerated in an educational establishment that tends to promulgate claims to knowledge that I refute, I forge Black feminist frameworks.

It is evident from Black women's descriptions of our gender and racial identities that myths about our sexuality circumscribe our lives. The dominant image of Black female sexuality influences identity and experiences. For some Black women the issue of 'race' does not affect their own notions of sexual identity and subsequently is not regarded as significant to their relationships. Others discover that derogatory images are so strong that without community support they internalize them. On a different tack I want to mention Edward Said's excellent investigation of 'Orientalism as a Western style for dominating, restructuring, and having authority over the Orient' (1978: 3). I want to use Said's concept of the Orient being seduced by the process of orientalizing, to consider the ways in which images of Black women affect us. In the creation of separate identities as Others, Said maintains, the modern Orient participates in orientalizing. The Orient is seduced into an acceptance of the rightness of the West's version of things (ibid.). In view of the institutionalization of myths it is not astonishing that some Black women collude with and encourage them. Nevertheless most Black women reject negative images of our sexuality and instead show the importance of self-determined definitions.

The extent to which opinions about identity are diverse and contradictory is illustrated by the fact that several women adhere to different aspects of identification. Some women argue that 'race' does not influence their sexual identity whilst asserting that they resist racialized sexual imagery in their daily lives. As such, the articulation of self-identities is subject to change, hybridity and conflict (Rutherford 1990). Hilary Davies, a 54-year-old nurse, believes that in the past 'race' affected the way she saw herself sexually as well as her experiences. Although when she was younger 'race' determined Hilary's ideas about sexuality she now just takes people as they are, including herself. Maria Campbell, a 50-year-old catering assistant, and Yvonne Ayoka Wilson, a student who is 20, believe that images of Black female sexuality do not contribute to their sense of self. Instead they agree with Yvonne Stewart's description of the impact of 'race' upon her identity:

> 'I've never thought about it really in that context. I just see myself as a woman. Black doesn't really come into it. It never has really in general. It's a strange question for me because having been brought up here in this country, I know I'm Black and I'm very proud to be Black, but it's never bothered me. I've never thought about it in terms sexually or in any other way at all. I've just thought of myself as a woman period. . . . These images don't affect me in the slightest in any form or fashion. I just see myself as a person. I don't really think about my colour too much because this is what I was born with and this is what I'm going to die with. . . . This is just me.'

Similarly Tammy Ryan, a 24-year-old housewife, and Bernice Watts, who is 30 and unemployed, stress that racialized sexual images do not influence their self-perceptions. Thus Bernice explains that:

> 'Sexual images about Black women don't affect me because I believe that I am who I am and nothing is going to change who I am.'

These views problematize the ways in which debates on identity tend to explain people's sense of 'who they are' in terms of either the internalization or the rejection of racial, gender and class divisions (ibid.). Moreover, the significance of being able to control what you are, what you want to be and what you want to become is explained as a negotiable process that is far more complicated than many theorists realize.

Consequently, Melisa thinks that the effects of images of Black women as sexual beings upon her own sense of self operate on different levels. On a primary level the image of Black women as hot and sexy, Melisa contends, does not influence her because she does not conform to it. However, the fact that she is aware of the image and actively tries to go beyond it suggests that it actually does have an important impact upon her identity. Nevertheless this awareness does not automatically signify resistance for she admits that sometimes, especially when she is depressed, she finds the image amusing and maybe even complimentary. Then she thinks 'I am a nice Black number' and projects a sensual image. Generally Melisa chooses not to live up to the label:

> 'I suppose I could take on that image of being a hot Black woman and I suppose my life would be totally different to how it is now. But because I don't, then I think it doesn't affect my life.'

This view is also supported by 45-year-old housewife Marva Taylor's assertion that:

> 'I see myself as being a sexual woman . . . I just see myself as an ordinary person.'

Susan Brown, a 28-year-old secretary, maintains that her perception of her sexual identity cannot be explained within the context of racism:

> 'I don't think colour matters in that respect. I think it's the way the person carries herself and how she respects herself. But colour, I can't see how it can affect a person. I think it's the individual. . . . Well I haven't really looked deep into myself as a Black woman. I just think neutral. If I do have to look at myself as a Black woman, I don't know, I don't see it as a colour issue. . . . As I'm getting older as well, now I'm getting neutral. I think you can think too much about colour on a day-to-day basis but I don't.'

Susan's notion of neutrality clearly supports the argument that the marginalization of Black women as the Other is integral to the formation of our identity (ibid.). Her notion of neutrality is actually one of refusing to see herself as a sexualized Black woman. I have shown that given the historical and ideological foundations of racialized sexual images it is necessary to query the degree to which a neutral position is indeed possible. Therefore I hope to explain that for Black women the articulation of identities is an inevitable, although maybe only at times conscious product of a gendered and racialized construction of our sexualities. As Jonathan Rutherford explains:

> Identity marks the conjuncture of our past with the social, cultural and economic relations we live within. . . . Making our identities can only be understood within the context of this articulation, in the intersection of our everyday lives with the economic and political relations of subordination and domination.
>
> (1990: 19–20)

The complex structuring of identities as contingent, displacing and subject to transformation is shown by Fiona Ferguson's description of the impact of stereotypes about Black women's sexuality:

> 'You try and ignore the stereotype. You make it clear that the stereotype isn't right. That's what I do. . . . These images don't affect me because I ignore them; because I think they're the wrong images. So I go out of my way to make it known that they are the wrong images. They affect me in that I'm conscious of them, and I make sure that I don't get viewed in that way, and I don't pander to them in any shape or form. . . . It doesn't affect me because of my attitude towards it and the attitudes of people that I meet/fuck.'

Some Black women, having been stigmatized by racialized sexual images in society generally and within Black communities, begin to internalize these images themselves. In relation to the force of common-sense ideas about Black sexuality and their reinforcement by institutions such as the mass media a minority of Black women comply to the myths. Roseanne argues that without strong support networks and with institutionalized racist and sexist stereotypes against them it is not surprising that a few Black women accept the mythology:

'There's nothing to help the Black woman to challenge these stereotypes. She's left eventually believing them herself; believing deep down that maybe we are rampant sex maniacs. . . . We've taken on board these stereotypes because we've had to accept certain images about ourselves by virtue of the way our lives are restricted by stereotypes that are not resistant to change. To challenge them actively in the way that actually rebukes what they're saying we can't; because they hold the key; they're in a position. We can't obtain the key. We can reach the key but the key is on the highest step and with that key you can open the doors and go anywhere that you want.'

The pervading force of external definitions of Black womanhood and the suppression of identity to which this gives rise is analysed by Audre Lorde. She criticizes the internalization of negative portrayals of Black women's sexuality because it makes us docile, loyal and obedient and as such accept our subordination:

When we live outside ourselves, and by that I mean on external directives only rather than from our internal knowledge and needs, when we live away from those erotic guides from within ourselves, then our lives are limited by external and alien forms, and we conform to the needs of a structure that is not based on human need, let alone an individual's.

(1984: 58)

Isolated from what we can be other than our social construction, some Black women not only internalize these images but actually put them forward as well. This is a way of taking power away from the image. Zora shows how Black women empower themselves in relation to negative imagery by counteracting the mythology of the bad Black mother/whore:

'You can't be anything else. I think a lot of Black women have taken those things and then they think OK, we can't define ourselves out of it so we are going to be the best there is. Either we are going to be the best mothers or we are going to be the best sexual beings or if we can manage it we'll be the best mothers and the best sexual beings.'

Due to strong images and the constraints of societal expectations it is extremely difficult for Black women to develop a

positive sense of self. Moreover the fear of exclusion and the need to feel accepted leads some Black women to conform to dominant myths. Fosuwa believes that:

> 'You are not allowed to say "look I'm just being". It goes to the myth of Black women and how they see Black women's sexuality. It's like she will always have somebody and if you don't want somebody it's like there's something drastically wrong with you. . . . Until you conform. . . . It makes people carry a lot of mental luggage.'

Furthermore Fosuwa argues that Black women often collude with dominant images and thereby encourage them. For instance, the way in which Black women dress and behave often has a hidden agenda. Hence Fosuwa suggests:

> 'Sometimes we collude in that because we haven't taken the myths on board. Sometimes Black women actually encourage, maybe subconsciously, a part of the myth-making.'

Supporting this point Beverley thinks that frequently Black women see ourselves as men's servants and so allow ourselves to be used as objects of sexual gratification. Beverley believes that we have to reject myths and to develop our own self-concepts:

> 'You have to first love yourself before you can love anybody. If a lot of women would take control of themselves and of their bodies, and everything else men would respect them. But women don't respect themselves so men would not respect them either; and I think that's the problem. . . . I think 'white' people paint a picture and we allow it to stick.'

In a similar way, in *The Beauty Myth*, Naomi Wolf explains that women are the slaves of our own bodies. We are entrapped in a beauty myth and if we are unable to achieve it we hate ourselves. Women's identity is premised upon European concepts that equate beauty with 'whiteness' and as such exclude Black women. The portrayal of women as virtuous beauties who are refined, pure, delicate, modest and physically frail supports the economic system:

> An economy that depends on slavery needs to promote images of slaves that 'justify' the institution of slavery. Western economies are absolutely dependent now on the continued under-

> payment of women. An ideology that makes women feel 'worth less' was urgently needed to counteract the way feminism had begun to make us feel worth more. This does not require a conspiracy; merely an atmosphere. The contemporary economy depends right now on the representation of women within the beauty myth.
>
> (Wolf 1990: 18)

Whilst it is important to realize that some Black women internalize and collude with controlling images it is fallacious to argue that they are consequently the willing participants in their own oppression. Nonetheless it is true that: 'A system of oppression draws much of its strength from the acquiescence of its victims, who have accepted the dominant image of themselves and are paralysed by a sense of helplessness.' (Murray 1987: 106)

As Black women we do not define ourselves in terms of racist sexual images but struggle to deconstruct and so reject them. Of course this is not to deny that stereotypes of Black female sexuality restrict Black women's lives socially, economically and politically in ways that are frequently difficult to reject. Accordingly Fosuwa explains that 'race' affects her sexual identity:

> 'Yes I think it does for any Black woman regardless of what your sexual preference is. Society does not let you forget because of the myths about Black women's sexuality. It's either ignored or you're supposed to be this exotic woman who can't have enough sort of image. So I think it does. It certainly does for me in terms of who I have relationships with, 'white' or Black.'

In spite of the obstacles most Black women recognize the falsity of images of Black womanhood and have discovered self-affirmation, strength and creative power through rejecting them. As the notion of identity is fluid there are a range of possibilities for change beyond the realm of imagery. This includes our incorporation into systems of power. A good example of this is the work of Black women artists, writers and film-makers who defy stereotypes and celebrate Black woman power. Thereby we change our identities as victims of oppression so that we actively resist our subordination. By challenging such images Black women are empowered to define and to be ourselves. Thus Sally states:

'In this country you also need to take into consideration the negative views about Black women and sexuality portrayed in the media; the television, the radio and in the papers. So in that respect you're constantly fighting against what is being portrayed; and you constantly say "look I'm a Black woman and I'm not a sexual animal." '

Part of this rejection entails projecting oneself in a way that negates the myths. Thus many Black women tend not to display their sexual side and so attempt to disprove the images. Fiona argues:

'I go out of my way to negate the image. . . . I think you go away thinking this is the image I've got on TV, or I'm portrayed in the media or in advertising and it's not true. Therefore it has to be made clear that it's the wrong image. . . . If the image is that Black women are easy then Black women aren't easy. You make sure that you don't let people think that you're easy. If you think that someone has got the image of a Black woman then you make sure that you don't pander that image. If you meet someone and you think that this person thinks that I am a Black woman, and I fall into this category according to the TV image, then you make sure that they realize that it is the wrong image.'

The victorious creation of Black women's identities in and for themselves is examined by Pratibha Parmar. Acknowledging that 'Black British women are part of many diasporas' (1990) she analyses our historical and cultural situation. Parmar assesses the articulation of positive Black female identity within the racist and sexist background of displacement, alienation and 'Otherness'. Thus Black women's situation of marginality and resistance is a site of both individual and collective radical identity. Parmar discusses the necessity of getting rid of binary oppositions because of the polarization of positive and negative categories:

This entails creating identities as Black British women not 'in relation to', 'in opposition to', 'as reversal of', or 'as a corrective' . . . *but in and for ourselves.* Such a narrative thwarts that binary hierarchy of centre and margin: the margin refuses its place as 'Other'.

(Parmar 1990: 101, emphasis in original)

Black women refute negative images about our sexuality and construct a positive self-definition not just for the benefit of identification but rather as a precursor to activism. We stress the revolutionary potential of Black women defining ourselves and maintain that this is a right that historically has been denied to us. We defy the ways in which definitions of Black womanhood have been determined by 'white' people and by Black men and argue that Black women's sense of self, our aspirations and conduct, have been restricted by external definitions of Black female sexuality. We assert that when Black women claim our sexuality as our own for no-one else to pass judgement on; this consciousness can lead to sexual autonomy. For instance Zora discusses how Black women's own definitions of our sexuality are integral to wider struggles for Black women's equality. Zora thinks that:

> 'It's to define yourself. I think that the most powerful thing that you can do is to define yourself; because so much definition has been done to us by other people; and then even our Black male counterparts can use you as something to define themselves against. None of that any more. The time has come. If they don't like it well tough. You've just got to keep on going and don't let anybody stand in your way. . . . Standing on your own two feet and on your own terms; and doing what you want to do, because that's the only way that things are going to change.'

Yet awareness of identification also needs to incorporate a critical self-evaluation of an individual's diverse personal and political personalities (see Rutherford 1990). Hence the independence and connections between 'race', class, gender and sexuality in the construction of our identities and experiences needs to be realized (ibid.). Surviving and opposing dominant ideological impositions we create and preserve unique cultural identities. Yvonne Stewart asserts the importance of fighting against racial and sexual stereotypes:

> 'I am a Black woman but look at me. I am Black yes but I can do a hundred per cent better than you. My skin is Black but it's not holding me back. . . . A Black woman is a Black woman. She can do anything she wants. She's a woman and that's what she should know. Number one she's a woman. She

can do it because we women are mainstay. We keep the world going.'

The power of self-definition as a means for Black women's rejection of externally defined images is shown by Patricia Hill Collins. She explains how Black women resolve the contradictions between controlling images and our daily experiences. Hence, Black women demystify the stereotypes and define ourselves. Moreover Black women's empowerment through self-definition enables us both to cope with and transcend our oppression. Collins asserts that:

> the controlling images applied to Black women are so uniformly negative that they almost necessitate resistance if Black women are to have any positive self-images. For Black women, constructed knowledge of self emerges from the struggle to reject controlling images and integrate knowledge deemed personally important, usually knowledge essential to Black women's survival.
>
> (Collins 1990: 95)

As I stated earlier self-definition is important as a precursor to structural change. Black women develop a secure sense of self, in which sexuality is not necessarily the most important issue. According to Fosuwa:

> 'My sexuality is very important to me. It's not the top of my list. I consider myself a Black lesbian feminist. A Black woman is much more important to me. It's not about who I sleep with. I mean that's the least of it and I sometimes wonder about people who make all of this gossip. That's not important at all times.'

Agreeing with this point, Zora explains how her own perception of her identity negates dominant images of Black female sexuality:

> 'The problem with Zora Day is that I don't see myself sexually first and foremost. . . . I'm a woman in which sex does not play a major role in my life although it does. It's kind of like a two-edged sword. It does when I want it to on my terms. . . . I suppose my sex is a very personal thing . . . and I suppose that is why I get annoyed when I think I'm clearly not being sexual, and it's almost as if "she's a woman, she's available,

we've just got to try it, she can't go by without us actually having a try." I'm not some damn horse you can break in.'

In stark contrast to sexual and racial stereotypes some Black women define themselves as respectable, faithful and religious. Both Patricia and Susan stress the significance of old-fashioned values. Patricia Ford, a 52-year-old nurse, purports that:

'Black women are close to their family. She gets married, brings up her children and tries to lead a decent quiet life. She goes out to work and brings in an honest pound to raise a decent family. She brings up her children in church. She takes them to Sunday school. She has a Christian mind. She doesn't have affairs because it's not her style. She tries to bring up her kids as nice and decent as can be.'

Susan adds:

'I believe in the family and family ties. I believe in marriage as well. I'm old-fashioned in that way.'

These views support Patricia Hill Collins' analysis of the importance of Black woman's independent self-definitions. Collins maintains that the journey from internalized oppression to the creation of positive identities is vital to challenging stereotypes. Furthermore:

Far from being a secondary concern in bringing about social change, challenging controlling images and replacing them with a Black woman's standpoint is an essential component in resisting systems of race, gender and class oppression.

(Collins 1990: 104)

The most central components to a progressive sense of self are seen as self-love, self-respect and independence. Beverley believes that:

'A woman first has to feel for herself. A woman first has to love herself.'

Bernice claims that:

'It's a feeling of self-worth. You have to know how much you want. You have to put forth a positive image, more so I feel at this particular time. And you can't let other people influence you because otherwise you aren't going to go forward.'

Zora stresses:

> 'Be your own person and you force them to accept you as you are. . . . We are who we are and we should be proud of who we are and to blazes with anybody else. And we are who we want to be.'

As Patricia Hill Collins argues, for Black women self-affirmation is created within the wider context of familial relations and Black communities. Consequently, self-esteem and self-respect necessarily entail demanding respect from others as well as respecting them. Moreover, self-valuation is also resourceful. A positive sense of self provides the assertiveness, self-reliance and independence that is pivotal to the liberation of Black women (Collins 1990). Indicating the force of being independent Beverley says:

> 'I see myself as an achiever. I see myself as an independent liberated woman. I know what I am and I know what I want.'

Fosuwa explains how an independent self-perception challenges stereotypes:

> 'so you have to go through a process of yourself throwing off some of those images. I walk deliberately. I take up space because I think I have a right to be in this world. I demand attention. For me that is a very positive thing to say "I am here; you will listen. If you won't listen then end of conversation"... "This is me as a Black woman". If you just think of me as sexual then that's your problem . . . I see myself as a very positive, strong Black woman.'

Believing that it is vital that we define ourselves, set our own agendas and control our lives we reject negative stereotypes. Through independent self-definitions we are empowered to know about ourselves and our lives in ways which transcend the limitations of racism, sexism, heterosexism and class oppression. A redefinition of Black female sexuality has to be incorporated into social policies so that the subordination of Black women, by virtue of attempts to control our sexuality, is challenged in concrete ways. Since equal opportunities policies are inadequately addressing the interface of 'race', gender and class in Black women's lives, a distinct critique of their links to oppression on the basis of sexuality does not seem imminent. Nevertheless, the onus is on us to force ideological, socioeconomic and political arenas such as the media, education, employment and housing to eradicate myths of Black female sexuality.

CONCLUSION

And still we rise! Interviewing these women has been a source of inspiration for me as I battle with my own simultaneous feelings of self-hate, anger, passion, respect and power. In spite of a history that militates against our progress, Black women strive to ameliorate our circumstances. The reasons for the continuance of negative stereotypes about our sexuality and the subjugation to which this gives rise is, as I have previously argued, inextricably linked to broader power relations. I must stress that contemporary British culture and economy to a large extent depend on the representation of Black women as hypersexual. Images of Black female sexuality have been used as a political weapon against the advancement of Black women in Britain. Although Black girls do relatively well at school, and as history shows us Black women have never been adverse to hard work, we are still on the lower echelons of the social structure. The inability of Black women to achieve our socioeconomic and political potentials has been institutionalized by the relegation of Black womanhood as being synonymous with rampant sexuality. Since we are only seen as sexual beings it is extremely difficult for us to gain social credence and power. The perpetuation of images of Black female sexuality constitutes a form of social control; a form of social coercion that attempts to undermine the status of Black women. If we give in to these images we become disillusioned, repressed and ultimately self-destructive.

Stereotypes of Black female sexuality prescribe behaviour for Black women that does more than disrupt our self-esteem, for they act as a justification for our subordination. Liberation from this situation entails new definitions of our sexualities. It is vital that these definitions are integrated into everyday ideas and practices. The women in this research have clearly demonstrated that self-identification is a means of counteracting controlling images. This can only transform the material position of Black women effectively when we unite and mobilize both autonomously and with supportive Black men and 'white' people to put the overthrow of racialized sexual imagery on the political agenda. In an increasingly conservative, racist, anti-feminist and homophobic environment the need for the ideological tools, the radical commitment, the revolutionary activism and the material resources to achieve our goals is pivotal. Beyond postmodern apathy is the possibility to recognize and organize around our commonalities and differences in relation to controlling images. So far an elite that is 'white', male, middle class and heterosexual has had the power to define and objectify groups as subordinate. The time has come for a new order. Those of us who have been marginalized must develop coalition politics that fight for the needs of Black women within the wider strategies of 'left-wing' groups, women's organizations, Black and gay movements.

ACKNOWLEDGEMENTS

With love to my parents -- Marlene and Doc Marshall. I especially thank Janice Acquah, Delia Jarrett-MacCauley, Karen McHugh, Rosemarie Mallett, Annie Phizacklea, Nigel Rudder and the women whom I interviewed for believing in me. For patiently helping me to move beyond my confusion whilst writing this essay I give 'nuff' respect to Andrea Massiah, Valentina Alexander and Julia Hallam.

BIBLIOGRAPHY

Bhabha, H. (1983) 'The other question – Homi K. Bhabha reconsiders the stereotype and colonial discourse', *Screen* 24(6): 18–36.
Bryan, B., Dadzie, S. and Scafe, S. (1985) *The Heart of the Race* London: Virago.
Bush, B. (1990) *Slave Women in Caribbean Society 1650–1838* Bloomington IN: Indiana University Press.
Collins, P. H. (1990) *Black Feminist Thought* London: Unwin Hyman.
Davis, A. (1982) *Women, Race and Class* London: Women's Press.
Donald, J. and Rattansi, A. (eds) (1992) *'Race', Culture and Difference* London: Sage.
Fanon, F. (1970) *Black Skin White Masks* London: Paladin.
Franklin, A. (1967) *I Never Loved a Man the Way I Love You* Atlantic Recording Corporation.
Fryer, P. (1988) *Black People in the British Empire* London: Pluto.
Gilman, S. (1985) *Difference and Pathology* Ithaca NY: Cornell University Press.
hooks, b. (1982) *Ain't I A Woman* London: Pluto.
Husband, C. (ed.) (1982) *'Race' in Britain* London: Hutchinson.
Jordan, J. (1989) *Moving Towards Home* London: Virago.

Jordan, W. D. (1982) 'First impressions: initial English confrontations with Africans' in C. Husband (ed.) *'Race' in Britain* London: Hutchinson.
Kovel, J. (1970) *White Racism* New York: Pantheon.
Lorde, A. (1984) *Sister Outsider* Freedom CA: The Crossing Press.
Murray, P. (1987) 'The liberation of black women' in M. L. Thompson (ed.) *Voices of the New Feminism* Boston: Beacon.
Parmar, P. (1990) 'Black feminism: the politics of articulation' in J. Rutherford (ed.) *Identity – Community, Culture, Difference* London: Lawrence & Wishart.
Rutherford, J. (ed.) (1990) *Identity – Community, Culture, Difference* London: Lawrence & Wishart.
Said, E. W. (1978) *Orientalism* London: Routledge & Kegan Paul.
Simmonds, F. N. (1988) 'She's gotta have it: the representation of black female sexuality on film' *Feminist Review* 29
Walker, A. (1981) 'Coming apart' *You Can't Keep a Good Woman Down* New York: Harcourt Brace Yovanovich.
Ware, V. (1992) *Beyond the Pale* London: Verso.
Wolf, N. (1990) *The Beauty Myth* New York: Vintage.
Young, L. (1990) 'A nasty piece of work: a psychoanalytic study of sexual and racial difference in "Mona Lisa" ' in J. Rutherford (ed.) *Identity – Community, Culture, Difference* London: Lawrence & Wishart.

Chapter 2

Exemplary women

Delia Jarrett-Macauley

INTRODUCTION

Among the papers of the African-American writer, activist and professor James Weldon Johnson is a long and friendly letter dated 27 January 1938 from a young Jamaican woman writer, Una Marson. This letter is very important to me because it reinforces the link between the distinguished Black American writers of the time and Una Marson, whose life-story I have been researching.[1] The letter's contents indicate that these writers were part of the same 'extended family' whose members prize identical great-grandparents, although the first cousins have never even swapped phone numbers. These writers, living in different parts of the African Diaspora, share several cultural concerns which are reflected in their work. So, in examining the life of Una Marson, an extraordinary Black West Indian woman, I have seen Caribbean writing and, to a lesser degree, some African-American writing, through a different lens.

In summer 1936, aged 31, Una Marson who had been living in England since 1932, returned to Jamaica. She found on her arrival, as any long-term exile must, that she had missed several events – some exciting and not likely to be repeated. Her friends and acquaintances, an eclectic group of writers, journalists, artists and activists, told her that they had recently entertained an African-American celebrity: Zora Neale Hurston. This anthropologist, novelist, folklorist and playwright, then in her late thirties, was visiting the British colony as part of a longer research trip to the West Indies during which she gathered folklore and material on Haitian 'voodoo'.[2]

In her letter of January 1938 to James Weldon Johnson, Una

Marson explained that Zora Neale Hurston had 'sailed away the very week of my return from London', so, sadly, these two never met. In their separate ways, however, Una Marson and Zora Neale Hurston were travelling the same path. Like Una, Zora spent her earliest years in a small, rural environment, a rich source of Black cultural traditions which she was to put to good use in her mature work. As an adult Zora, like Una, was said to be contradictory, and 'difficult'. They preferred to invent new ways of being rather than unthinkingly to follow the status quo. Both were drawn to men of intellectual quality: they needed and appreciated the critical perception of male literary figures such as James Weldon Johnson and, at different periods, Langston Hughes, with whom they could share their desire to have Black writing and cultural forms better known.[3] However in both their lives it was other women who provided the 'on-going fascination and sustenance of life' – practical, day-to-day support, family or a sense of belonging. (Rich 1986: 56) Zora Neale Hurston and Una Marson were apt to make huge leaps in creativity which their male peers and later critics did not altogether support. And both were doing their best to destroy hackneyed images of Black women in literature and society, by exploring relationships between women: mothers, daughters, sisters, or aunts.

Una Marson (1905–65) was a poet, playwright, journalist, broadcaster, publisher and social activist. She was the first West Indian female poet to explore the particular feelings and circumstances of the Black woman. Living in Jamaica during the 1920s, Una Marson had been conscious of the lack of professional and leisure opportunities available to women of her social class. She began to challenge gender conventions for both middle- and working-class women in her creative work and in her professional life, starting a union for secretaries, encouraging feminist action and writing about the 'New Woman'. In summer 1932 she travelled to England and became involved in various women's and Black political groups, working for the Ethiopian Legation during the 1935–36 Italian–Ethiopian war. When the war ended, in summer 1936 she returned to Jamaica.

By the time Zora Neale Hurston arrived in Jamaica in April 1936 she was already a celebrated artist of the Harlem Renaissance and had come to prominence through her representation of Black rural folk culture. She had produced three musicals, published the novel *Jonah's Gourd Vine* (1934), and short stories such as 'Sweat' – about a marriage that is torn apart through economic inequality – and 'The Gilded Six-Bits', as well as a collection of folklore tales from the rural south *Mules and Men* (1935). On her arrival in Kingston, *The Daily Gleaner*, Jamaica's leading paper, pictured her in 'jodpurs and riding garb, her hat at a rakish angle, ready for a sortie into the tropical bush'.

This two-year sortie, which included extensive work in Haiti, produced *Tell My Horse* (1938), an autobiographical work with extended sections on voodoo and Haitian politics. Although Robert Hemenway, her biographer, has dismissed this as 'Hurston's poorest book' (Hemenway 1986: 248), since her talents, he says, lay in other literary forms, not political analysis or travel writing, the first section, 'Jamaica', contains some interesting observations of the British colony by this Black intellectual. Indeed, we have far too few records of what Black women thought about their position in society, work, sexuality or culture, so although the book suffers from a somewhat romantic vision and is weakened by its American patriotic and imperial perspective, it remains a worthwhile testimony and (conveniently) brings Zora Neale Hurston into Una Marson's intellectual and geographical territory.

Had they met, Una and Zora might have taken to the hills of St Mary to chat and compare notes on writing, cultural politics, feminist and 'race' politics. Una would have taken her large black bag, stuffed with papers, poetry, scripts, play programmes and articles to show her visitor, and Zora would surely have taken off her hat and listened to Una's version of the way things were in Jamaica.

MAKING OURSELVES VISIBLE

What framework can comprehend both Una and Zora and allow us to see what they might have shared?

Simply to point out that they are both early twentieth-century Black women writers is to indicate a starting point. As Mary Helen Washington, writing about African-American women's literary tradition, has observed, there is:

> a single distinguishing feature of the literature of black women – and this accounts for their lack of recognition – it is this their literature is about black women; it takes the trouble

> to record the thoughts, words, feelings and deeds of black women . . .
>
> (Washington 1987: xxi)

Even today, literary historians of Caribbean writing have observed how rarely Black women appear as active subjects in Caribbean literature. This has occurred in spite of Black women's vital economic role since slavery. To grasp the significance of Zora and Una's writings on the Jamaican woman, it is worth casting back to her earlier appearances in the island's literature.

The small number of free 'white' women who resided in the West Indies during the years of slavery left a substantial body of written material about their domestic lives and travels, nostalgic thoughts of distant England. Among these historical sources there is the incomparable diary of Maria Nugent, the wife of the Governor of Jamaica from 1801 to 1805. Here Maria Nugent accords some space to her observations about Black women:

> Nelly Nugent remarked, however, that it was astonishing how fast these Black women bred, what healthy children they had, and how soon they recovered after laying-in. She said it was totally different with mulatto women, who were constantly liable to miscarry, and subject to a thousand little complaints, colds, coughs etc. Indeed, I have heard medical men make the same observation.
>
> (quoted in Gutzmore 1986: 29)

Mary Nugent, always an inquisitive woman, kept her diary diligently and, in the process, revealed much about the sexual mores of her class:

> I dressed and walked about the house till dinnertime. A little mulatto girl was sent into the drawing room to amuse me. She was a sickly delicate child, with straight light-brown hair, and very black eyes. Mr T. appeared very anxious for me to dismiss her, and in the evening, the housekeeper told me she was his own daughter, and that he had a numerous family, some almost on every one of his estates.
>
> (ibid.: 30)

Nowhere, needless to say, is the reader confronted with the full humanity of the Black woman slave since she is only 'chattel', her work a unit of labour, and her body a boon to her owner, or a bane if she is ill. The inner life of the slave woman or man is irretrievable without an imaginative leap on the part of the historian (see e.g. Brathwaite 1971). Twentieth-century Caribbean historians ranging from Kamau Brathwaite and Elsa Goveia to the younger generation, led by Lucille Mathurin, have added the emotional discourse to the slave's story, while conventional written sources – court records, estate documents, diaries of the planter class, Colonial Office and parliamentary reports – the official history of the slave person provide him or her with no 'voice'.

Mary Seacole is the only woman of colour whose voice breaks that long silence stretching from the end of slavery to the 1930s. Her autobiography, *Wonderful Adventures of Mary Seacole in Many Lands* which focuses on her work in the Crimean war, was published in London in 1857, and reissued in 1984 when Ziggi Alexander and Audrey Dewjee edited the forgotten classic. Mary Seacole, a 'female Ulysses' who 'remained an unprotected female' not out of necessity, but because she had confidence in her own powers, is an alternative voice countering the bourgeois ideology of what a Black woman should be (Alexander and Dewjee 1984: 14).

This dauntless business woman who learnt her medical skills from her mother, 'an admirable doctress', had practised on her dolls and pets before embarking on her profession:

> I was always a hearty, strong woman – plain-spoke people might say stout – I think my heart is soft enough.
>
> . . . My fortunes underwent the variations which befall all. Sometimes I was rich one day, and poor the next. I never thought too exclusively of money, believing rather that we were born to be happy, and that the surest way to be wretched is to prize it over-much. Had I done so, I should have mourned over many a promising speculation proving a failure, over many a pan of preserves or guava jelly burnt in the making.
>
> (ibid.: 58)

And yet, Mary Seacole's sense of freedom is impaired by the colour/class hierarchy of her island. She depicts herself defensively:

> I am a Creole, and have good Scotch blood coursing in my veins. . . . I have often heard the term 'lazy Creole' applied to

my country people; but I am sure I do not know what it is to be indolent.

(ibid.: 55)

Poor Mary, like Una Marson a century later, was born into a region in which the upper and middle classes, whether 'white'-skinned or not, were so oriented towards Europe that any defence against the myth of Black inferiority seemed almost inconceivable. The books which adorned their libraries were, in the main, English classics, the preferred sustenance of the colonized mind.

When the Jamaican writer Claude McKay who was resident in the United States for many years, turned his attention to such a 'native gentleman' in his novel *Banana Bottom* (1933), he described him as the owner of: 'one of the best houses in Jubilee [who] possessed a fine library where he entertained his friends. Beautifully bound Collected Works of Great British Authors. Novelists, Essayists, Poets in fine glass cases ranged round the walls'. But when Bita, the heroine, examined the collection volume by volume she discovered that the pages of every book were uncut. ' "But it's nice to furnish a room like this with fine books and bookcases. It is the fashion and gives distinction" said the "native gentleman".' (quoted in Sander 1978: 33–5)

Not every literate Jamaican was guilty of perpetrating such facade, yet many educated Black people, determined to show that colour is only skin-deep, preferred to have nothing to do with their African origins or the taint of slavery. An inevitable consequence was an eradication of Black imagery within accepted culture. It was only in the 1930s, when Edna Manley, the English-born Jamaican sculptor produced works such as 'Negro Aroused', that an African history began to be celebrated. The early twentieth century also saw the arrival of the 'virtuous', 'refined' Black woman in local literature in the writings of Constance Hollar and others. Here Hollar depicts her grandmother as a saint:

Hair brushed on either side her face
And such a look of quiet grace
In liquid eyes of brown
A bible open on her knee
It is thus I often see
My grandmother
My lovely little grandmother

This was a deliberate attempt to 'uplift the race', particularly to expunge the notion of the immoral Black woman, but such sentimental reframing failed to account for the Black, Black grandmothers – the slave women, daughters of slaves and mothers of working classes. These women were written out of the literature; their opinions and feelings were ignored as strongly in the post-emancipation period as they had been in slavery. In 1938, a century after emancipation, the masses of the people were landless, semi-literate and without the vote. That spring, despair at the seemingly endless inter-war depression, at the appalling lack of social facilities, low wages, insanitary housing and empty bellies led, inevitably, to fierce and bloody protest. The Mayor of Kingston, Oswald Anderson, caught that despair when he wrote:

> Poverty walks the island, and it is the first thing that is seen in our country. It is not because the people do not want work, but it is the working-man and the peasant farmer alike who are in the grip of dire poverty. . . . The boast in Kingston, now, is the establishment of a Food Depot for School Children, where they can obtain lunch at the rate of 1d a day, while no dog in the homes of the employers could be as miserably treated. There is plenty of want and it calls for plenty of pity.[4]

It is against this background that Zora and Una's observations of Jamaican women should be read. In rural parishes women still worked the land, growing citrus fruits, bananas, and coffee; in the city they were employed breaking stones, loading coal at the harbour or as domestics, washing and cleaning for the wealthy. Zora Neale Hurston and Una Marson brought these women to life in their works, recognizing that they were more than mere units of labour whose existence helped or hindered the economic viability of the newfangled plantation:

> In Jamaica it is common sight to see skinny-looking but muscular black women sitting on top of a pile of rocks with a hammer making little ones out of big ones. They look so wretched with their bare black feet all gnarled and distorted from walking barefooted over rocks. The nails on *their big toes thickened like a hoof* from a life time of knocking against stones. All covered over with the gray dust of the road, those feet look almost saurian and repellent.
>
> (Hurston 1938: 58, emphasis added)

This, one of the few contemporary descriptions of how some of the poorest, dark-skinned, Black women – those who bore the brunt of class, colour and gender oppressions – earned their living was offered as evidence that 'women get no bonus just for being female down there'. It foreshadows Hurston's most striking metaphor, 'de mule uh de world', used in the later novel *Their Eyes Were Watching God* and throughout her work. For instance, Janie (the heroine of *Their Eyes*) empathically comments: 'People ought to have some regard to helpless things'.

For Una Marson also the image of the stonebreakers answered the search for an authentic literary code that would expose the harshness of Jamaica's socioeconomic hierarchy to its complacent bourgeoisie. Her representation of these women labourers takes the form of a private, sisterly dialogue through which their arduous lives are contrasted with the idle pursuits of their men: 'Dem wutless pupa tan round de bar/A trow dice de day'. As in much of Una Marson's writing, these women find solace and security with one another; they seem to create a haven where neither 'backra' ('white' boss), nor family, nor lover, can intrude:

Liza me chile, I's really tired
Fe broke dem stone
Me han hat me
Me back hat me
Me foot hat me
An lard de sun a blin me

No so, Cousin Mary, an den
De big Backra car dem
A lik up de dus in a we face
Me massa jesus know it
I's weary of dis wol' –

But whey fe do, Cousin Mary
Me haf fe buy frack fe de pickney dem
Ebry day dem had fe feed
Dem wutless pupa tan round de bar
A trow dice all de day
De groun is dat dry
Not a ting will grow –
Massy Lard, dis life is hard
An so – dough de work is hard

I will had to work fe pittance
Till de good Lard call me

Liza chile, I's really tired
But wha fe do – we mus brok de stone
Dough me han dem hat me
Me back it hat me
An de sun it blin me
Well – de good Lard knows
All about we sorrows

(Marson, 'Stonebreakers' 1937)

By the time Una Marson and Zora Neale Hurston published these vignettes of Jamaican women stonebreakers, the emancipation of the slaves was reaching its centenary. Too little had improved in the material condition of Black women's lives between 1838 and 1938. In pre- and post-emancipation Jamaica, occupation denoted a person's social status. The New World plantation had been organized primarily towards a single economic goal, with both a racial and sexual division of labour. While men could be employed as carpenters, masons, blacksmiths, fishermen, wheelwrights, sawyers and so on, women almost always worked in the fields, in gangs, or as domestics. 'One is struck' writes historian Orlando Patterson, 'by the fact that male slaves had a much wider range of occupation to choose from than females: apart from being domestics and fieldhands, the latter could only be washerwomen, cooks and nurses' (1967). Come the end of slavery, there was nothing some women and men wanted more than to be gone from the plantation. But what to do? While the skilled male worker could have set himself up in trade, enjoyed some (little) status, greater comfort and job satisfaction; the woman, unskilled, untrained, and in surplus numbers, suffered job degradation. With no easy avenue to respect, independence or comfort, she either remained as a domestic or field hand or found herself loading coal or breaking stone. Her work status immediately denoted a particular social niche. The severity of the stonebreaker's job – today often associated with hard labour in male prisons – said it all.

PATHWAYS TO DESTRUCTION: 'RACE', SEXUALITY AND GENDER ENTRAPMENTS

> Friday 22nd May 1752. At about 4pm Heard a gun go off behind the Negro houses. Upon enquiry found it was fired by John Filton. Immediately went to look for him, but not finding him searched Phibbah's house, and there found him hid upon her bed beyond the door, in pretended sleep. Discharged him [from] the plantation before Mr Samuel Mordiner. Note, a Mulatto, and one or more Negro men with him. Had Phibbah directly given about 70 lashes for harbouring him in her house.
>
> (Thistlewood, quoted in Hall 1989)

This account of jealousy, fear and punishment is from the diary of Thomas Thistlewood (1720–86). The second son of a Lincolnshire farmer, he arrived in Jamaica in 1750 and became overseer on the Egypt estate in Westmoreland the following year. He had a long-standing, but turbulent relationship with Phibbah who later became his 'wife' and mother of one of his sons. As the slave woman in charge of the cook room in the Great House, Phibbah had access to information about Thistlewood's employer, his other employees and slaves – a position which made her potentially influential among slaves and vulnerable to her master. (John Filton, Thistlewood's predecessor at Egypt estate, may also have been a source of information to Phibbah.)

The sexual relationship between Phibbah and Thistlewood was, needless to say, commonplace. Sexual relations between planter-class men and slave women were part of the divide and rule technique of the owners, who regarded any woman of colour, Black or brown, as fair game for their pleasure and profit (see e.g. Brathwaite 1969; Patterson 1967). Sexual violence, rape, concubinage and other forms of exploitation and degradation were neither illegal nor frowned upon, except by a negligible minority. Stable sexual unions and motherhood were discouraged among slaves, so brief relationships became customary, although motherhood was treated with respect in slave communities. Slave women used every means at their disposal to protect their young. In Port Royal in the 1820s, for example, several women at Orchard Plantation – Dido, Rosetta, Lizzy, Augusta and Tuba – complained to the magistrates that their masters had directed their children to be taken from them and weaned from the breast, although the infants were too young to be left. When the magistrates investigated their complaint they found the infants were at least 'a twelve months old each, the women were reprimanded and directed to proceed back to the property to work' (quoted in Mathurin Mair 1975: 16–17).

After emancipation these social patterns changed only slightly. There were more marriages among free Blacks, but women preferred to live independently, taking money from their children's fathers as and when it was available, but otherwise caring for their families and themselves in closely knit communities. Bourgeois men of all racial groups resented autonomous working women whose lifestyles made a mockery of their ideals of chaste, domestic womanhood. As the Jamaican literary critic Rhonda Cobham has shown, the lower-class working woman came to be seen as unusually industrious and sexually promiscuous. The working woman's lifestyle, an affront to Victorian morality, was condemned as sinful and unchaste. And yet, her industry could not be overlooked. It is not surprising therefore that several early twentieth-century novels were preoccupied with this social realism. Most resolved the inner contradiction by playing off the woman's independent spirit against her sexual and economic needs, and so discrediting her (see Cobham-Sander 1980: 201).

Throughout their writings, Zora Neale Hurston and Una Marson are preoccupied with the interface of 'race'/sexuality/gender, and their attempts to explore this in Jamaica bear some comparison. In *Tell my Horse* Zora recounts a tale about a pretty brown-skinned young woman from a rural parish who comes to Kingston to work, is seduced by a fellow brown-skinned man on the eve of his wedding to another woman, and then unceremoniously dumped. A year or two later, having heard that this woman was to be married, the man told of his own experience with her and asked her prospective husband, 'You don't want second-hand goods do you?'. The other man did not and so she was again rejected.

Una Marson's early writing is dominated by the theme of lonely, rejected women for whom the supreme goal of marriage remains elusive. Throughout her early verse she depicts women characters who, like the woman in Zora's anecdote, are deemed by society to be sexually undesirable by men. The woman may be too dark-skinned, or she may attempt an inter-racial relationship; she may try to be submissive, sweet and pure, while she would prefer to be independent, powerful and valuable. Whatever the cause, the woman is always rejected by men in the end and left asking:

Question

Why can't you love me dearly
As other lovers do?

If

If you can love and not make love your master,
If you can serve yet do not be his slave,
If you can hear bright tales and quit them faster
And for your peace of mind, think him no knave.

(Marson 1930: 50, 83)

The only conclusion that can be drawn from Una Marson's many poetic investigations into the question of heterosexual love for educated Black Jamaican women is that it is both unlikely and debilitating.

In *Their Eyes Were Watching God* Zora Neale Hurston was to depict a passionate, deep and serious love affair between two Black people. Nothing of this emotional quality surfaces in Jamaican literature of that period. Una showed how the disappointment of romantic love could be healed, but she refrained from suggesting that a fuller, more generous love was attainable. Sexual fulfilment eludes the Black middle-class Jamaican woman just as true economic independence eludes her. Her lack of sexual freedom and autonomy act as a metaphor for her wider experience. In *At What a Price* (1931), Una Marson's first play, the Black country-born woman who migrates to the city for work is championed. The heroine, Ruth Maitland, enjoys and benefits from female companionship but her relationship with a 'white' foreigner leads only to disgrace and disappointment, compelling her to return to the circumscribed rural world she had once escaped.

The forced happy ending does not diminish the political impact of the play which airs questions about sex in a racialized context bravely and effectively. Una confronted the issue of colour prejudice in sexual relations and drew attention to the tendency of Jamaican men to marry upward on the colour scale. These issues are still relevant today, as evidenced in Sistren's theatre company's book *Lionheart Gal: Life Stories of Jamaican Women*. In the introduction they describe sexuality and motherhood as central to the experience of womanhood, adding:

> In all cases both the act of sex and becoming a mother are experienced as processes which heighten women's alienation from the societies they are supposed to be a part of. Sex is neither pleasurable nor empowering. It is indeed the pathway to destruction since through it women lose whatever tenuous possibility of autonomy they may have had.
>
> (1986: xix)

CULTURAL CONSERVATORS

Una and Zora's approaches to Jamaican life were distinct, but they shared a fundamental belief that the island's unofficial history – the folk history which remained on the island in the lives, customs, stories, songs, markets, rituals and memories of the people – needed to be rediscovered and dignified. Zora Neale Hurston represented this folk consciousness in her collection of folklore tales *Mules and Men* and later in *Their Eyes Were Watching God*.

In Kingston Zora heard about the religious form pocomania (said to mean 'a little crazy') and appreciated that its wide practice among the people made it worthy of scrutiny. She also loved her people's culture and saw beauty and wisdom in it. At home in the United States Zora had chosen to use her academic training to conserve and communicate what had been dismissed and disregarded even by the intellectual elites of her country and 'race'. As Hemenway writes her training with anthropologist Franz Boas 'provided more than an explanation for Eatonville's [Zora's home town] existence. It revealed how folklore could be served without transformation into conscious art' (1986: 81). Her work in the West Indies extended that project beyond the geographical/national boundaries of home.

Pocomania, Una Marson's third play, can be seen as an imaginative conservation and reinterpretation of Jamaican folk culture. The play, first produced in Kingston in January 1938 during the heyday of the nationalist movement, struck all contemporary critics as a genuine beginning of national theatre because its subject-matter, language and characters were all recognizably Jamaican. At last, Jamaican drama resembled Jamaican life. The conservative education which had taught Una Marson to denigrate that local eclecticism did not finally prevent her from becoming a cultural conservator of her times.

Zora and Una, these guardians of 'discredited knowledge' gave cultural meaning to Jamaican independence many years before the political reality arrived.[5] As women of African descent they both felt a strong, organic if discontinuous link with the struggle to keep African cultural connections and reconnections alive. They also believed that the various forms of cultural imperialism which had ruled both America and the West Indies should be put firmly in their place. They were engaged in reinventing a new cosmology through reassessing, reworking the African/slave/folk past.

Their range of literary genres was significant. Both writers chose to represent Black life through creative works and non-fiction alike – journalism, reportage, anthropology, biographical writings and essays. These genres enabled them to reconcile hard evidence with interpretation. Without each author physically distancing herself from her domestic source, these intellectual works would not have been produced. It is little wonder then that both grew intellectually by travelling extensively and crossing multiple boundaries, refusing to allow the elites of their 'race' or the constraints of gender or class to dictate their politics. In *Mules and Men*, Zora Neale Hurston explains:

> It was only when I was off in college, away from my native surroundings, that I could see myself like somebody else and stand off and look at my garment. Then I had to have the spy-glass of Anthropology to look through that.
>
> (1990: 17)

Although Una Marson did not claim the vantage point of an academic discipline, physical distance and extensive reading gave her a spy-glass for viewing Jamaican cultural forms and cultural production as well as the respectability her audience looked for. As a well-travelled intellectual, she represented in her person the transformation of a village child into a modern cosmopolitan woman. Una Marson knew how quickly traditions could be lost and called on Jamaicans to guard their own history and tell their own stories:

> We have it on the authority of no less a person than Aldous

> Huxley that in Europe and America twenty thousand million pounds of wood pulp and esparto grass are annually blackened with printers ink; the production of newspapers takes rank in many countries, among the major industries; in English, French and German alone, forty thousand new books are published every year. . . . I think I can say quite fairly, even without a complete list of Jamaican publications, that the intelligentsia of Jamaica do not realise the importance of literature to a country.
>
> (Marson 1937b)

The contemporary West Indian intellectual C. L. R. James, the activist, historian and political theorist, was also able through travel, study and political activism to review Caribbean history, and his work was also multi-faceted. His novel *Minty Alley* (1936) pushed at the boundaries of West Indian fiction by introducing the 'yard' life of poor city people. This novel, 'a major forerunner of the Caribbean literary movement in English, which has flourished mainly after 1950' (Elliot Parris 1986), was however only one part of James's Caribbean cultural project. James went further in his more overtly political work *The Black Jacobins* (1938) – the first full thesis on slave rebellion which was to have profound international impact within a Pan-African context. James was able to record what a profound, international impact this work had had; in his Foreword to the 1980 edition James wrote:

> I was tired of reading and hearing about Africans being persecuted and oppressed in Africa, in the Middle Passage, in the USA and all over the Caribbean. I made up my mind that I would write a book in which Africans and people of African descent instead of constantly being the object of other people's exploitation and ferocity would themselves take action on a grand scale and shaping other people to their own needs.

I wish to suggest, given that Black women's intellect is so often underestimated, that both Zora and Una were establishing new contours of *knowledge*, just as James was. Their work made the private autonomous domain of Black women's lives and Black cultural expression significant, and carried transformative power.

By reinterpreting history, culture, religious practice and Black women's lives, Una Marson and Zora Neale Hurston were engaging in revolutionary acts. If Black women are not victims, sapphires, whores and fools, then the whole world is different. In *Pocomania* Una Marson's female protagonist is aware that Western, Christian doctrine is not for her and does not serve her life: she forms her closest alliance with a 'woman of the people', Sister Kate whose strength comes from her slave, African, woman-centred culture. Similarly Zora Neale Hurston's *Mules and Men*, a collection of stories, voodoo rituals, songs and proverbs, creates different ways of seeing, different languages which carry aesthetic as well as social messages. And in *Their Eyes Were Watching God*, the celebrated character Janie lives by her own rules and the advice of her grandmother, rather than that of male-dominated society.

In these, their major works, Zora and Una present a critique of marriage and other institutions that can inhibit women's self-actualization, and they question the ideals of male superiority. The usual heterosexual couple is supplanted for other, same-sex relationships between mother and daughter, sisters, or aunts. Their female protagonists' highly developed imagination and sensitivity enable them to envisage a self-determined life-style and to counter the restrictions they have experienced in their formative years.

SAVING THE PRECIOUS AND PRECOCIOUS SPIRITS

Any form of literary or cultural history which attempts to pit one Black woman writer against another, or to suggest that a group which has so often been subject to unfair criticism, derision and exclusion can find its future in structuring a hierarchy of greatest suffering would be repugnant. But let it be said that in some respects in 1936 Una and Zora were very different, beyond personal characteristics of course.

The context of their writing lives differed sharply. Zora had received funding (though not without compromise) from her 'white' American patron, Mrs Mason, and from the Guggenheim Foundation for her research in the Caribbean. Looked at from the perspective of an under-resourced, unfunded West Indian young woman, like Una, this was a striking example of the importance of practical resources and their ability to facilitate creative and scholarly innovation. Although she had not come from a wealthy family, Zora Neale Hurston had studied at

Howard University, a Black school, for seven years, and later at Bernard College. She had access to resources which would have struck any contemporary West Indian artist and thinker as superior. For in Jamaica, as in the rest of the British West Indies, there were no universities – Black or otherwise. Indeed, when Una Marson was born in Jamaica there were no publishing houses, hardly any bookshops, critics, writers or libraries; no Guggenheim Foundation, no literary magazines. There was no question of Una Marson or women of her ilk simply joining in emergent Black literary circles – these still had to be created. There was almost no cultural scaffolding to hold on to; it had to be built.

What can such difference signify? It must point to the often disavowed truth about life in the British colonies during the first part of this century. It also indicates some of the differences between the African-American and African-Caribbean (female/literary) traditions. The Black writers of the colonies worked in an environment which was politically intolerant, educationally deprived and economically stagnant. Such contexts, whether in Port of Spain, Trinidad or Port Royal, Jamaica would scarcely favour vibrant Black female expression.

Today the reemergence of the African-Caribbean woman's past depends to some extent on the existence of archives, academic institutions and accessible sources which perceive Black women's history as vital to the region as a whole. But since higher education establishments are relatively new and public archives are facing tough economic crises, the African-Caribbean woman's voice cannot easily be heard. Some of the difficulties of reconstructing her past have been documented by Jamaican historian Lucille Mathurin Mair, to whom this chapter owes much. In *Recollections of a Journey into a Rebel Past* (1990) she writes about the pioneer publication of Caribbean women, *Savacou* 13, a special women's issue of the journal of the Caribbean Arts Movement, which she edited in 1977. This edition was remarkable for its inclusion of historical and contemporary materials, its multi-disciplinary shaping and its acknowledgement of the region's oral and written traditions. Edward Kamau Brathwaite dedicated *Savacou* 13 to Una Marson, whom Lucille Mathurin Mair terms a 'precious and precocious spirit', like her own foremother Nanny of the Maroons and other (slave) rebel Jamaican women. Una Marson, she writes:

> would have been at home with her wayward ancestors, those fractious females who ridiculed their masters, downed their tools, harassed the courts, placed themselves between their children and the slave driver, refused to give birth on order, planted their food crops, walked ten miles to market, flaunted their bright finery, and disappeared in the melting pot of towns, where they joined the men in plotting poison, arson and rebellion.
>
> (Mathurin Mair 1990: 59)

Some Caribbean writers and artists are engaged in exploring this wide circle of Black women's history and literary history, both within the region and throughout the metropoles of the former colonial and neo-colonial countries. Sometimes women's lives have not been recorded because they had 'no official voice of recognised history', as in the case of Elma Francois, the St Vincentian activist of the 1930s (see Busia 1991).

In the United Kingdom the lives of Mary Seacole and Claudia Jones have been recorded and there are now various local attempts to safeguard oral testimonies.

Almost all of this work goes on outside the academy, unlike in the United States. British academics have shown little interest in their former Black colonial subjects whether in the colonies or in Britain itself. As Ziggi Alexander writes:

> In the absence of a systematic and continuous tradition of Black historical research in the United Kingdom the search for primary source material in the form of letters, diaries, autobiographies, testimonies, photographs and drawings, is an important step in the process of reclaiming Black women's history. How much of value has been lost because white historians are reluctant to accept that contributions valid for interpretation have been made by Black people, particularly women? How many more Black women are there whose histories, thoughts, words and images remain buried in our archives?
>
> (Alexander 1988)

As the works of a migrant people, Caribbean women's writing benefits from a critical focus which cuts across geographic boundaries and is wary of rigid national compartmentalization. The value of such a framework enhances the reading of Paule Marshall, Audre Lorde, Jamaica Kincaid, Rosa Guy and Michelle Cliff – Caribbean-Americans – as much as it does of their American-born counterparts.

As world travellers Zora and Una were both able to write about Black women's experiences from various countries including the United States, England, Jamaica and Haiti. Not surprisingly the writing of such women who moved between countries and cultures was not always respected or understood by their critics. For example, as Mary Helen Washington has described, Zora Neale Hurston was caricatured by Wallace Thurman, devalued by Darwin Turner and dismissed by leading Harlem Renaissance critic Nathan Huggins. Meanwhile, Una Marson was accused of insincerity by fellow Jamaican poet, Clare McFarlane and patronized by newspaper editor and novelist Herbert G. Delisser. As late as 1968, only the most conservative literary tastes of the Caribbean poets were being canonized by Western critics (see e.g. James 1968). During the 1970s the ground was prepared for the recognition of these writers through the establishment of feminist literary criticism within the academy, and the emergence of culturally specific forms of evaluating Black texts such as the interest in oral story-telling traditions. Finally the early 1980s brought perceptive and detailed studies of African-American and African-Caribbean women writers. Only the tenacity and esteem of Black writers provided the critical methods that would serve the foremothers' art and intellect.

In the end the lives of Una Marson and Zora Neale Hurston can scarcely fail to strike us as comparable. These kindred artistic spirits, both committed writers, although subject to unfair criticism, long-term exclusion from the canon, misrepresentation and belittlement, have reemerged from our archives. They both died in late middle age. They had completed their major works, the texts for which they are now remembered, during their thirties and forties. And in later life each suffered personal sorrows which turned her creative force away from the literary world as she grew older. Una and Zora could not have known, though they might have guessed, that each would be relegated to the archives of literary history for much longer than their talents or output warranted. Una Marson had transformed representations of Jamaican women in poetry and in her plays. She was a pioneer of her time, in search of a cultural politics that would serve the African-Caribbean experience, by using nation language and reflecting the long-neglected voices of the people. Zora Neale Hurston had used anthropology to serve African-Americans and to assert the right of Black women to self-actualization.

Both Zora and Una were curious about each other's world, what lay between them and how they might differ. Their travels and subsequent writings gave form and imagination to the notions of international sisterhood and Black feminisms. They died before they could see what an impact such works might have on the next generation. But between them lay the literary possibilities for women of the African Diaspora in the late twentieth century.

NOTES

1 The biography of Una Marson (1905–65) is unpublished.
2 'Voodoo' is the term usually used; it is derived from 'vodun'.
3 The letters of both women to James Weldon Johnson reveal their desire to make Black culture and artists known. See for example, Zora Neale Hurston to James Weldon Johnson, 8 May 1934, where she says of the *New York Times*' review of *Jonah's Gourd Vine* that she 'never saw such a lack of information about us'.
4 Anderson to Harold Moody, 5 July 1938, Creech Jones Papers, 25/1.
5 The term is Toni Morrison's. See *Black Women Writers* (ed.) Evans, M. (London: Pluto Press, 1984).

BIBLIOGRAPHY

Alexander, Z. (1988) 'Black entertainers 1900–1910', *Feminist Arts News*, 2(5): 6–8.
Alexander, Z. and Dewjee, A. (eds) (1984) *The Wonderful Adventures of Mary Seacole in Many Lands*, London: Falling Wall Press.
Anderson, O. (1938) Letter to Harold Moody, 5 July, Creech Papers 25/1.
Awkward, M. (ed.) (1990) *New Essays on* Their Eyes Were Watching God, Cambridge and New York: Cambridge University Press.
Brathwaite, E. K. (1969) *The Development of Creole Society in Jamaica 1770–1820*, Oxford: Clarendon Press.
Brathwaite, E. K. (1971) *The Folk Culture of Slaves*, London and Port of Spain: New Beacon Books.
Brathwaite, E. K. (1974) *Contradictory Omens: Cultural Diversity and Integration in the Caribbean*, Kingston: Savacou Publications.
Busia, A. P. (1991) 'Rebellious women: fictional biographies' in S. Nasta (ed.) *Motherlands*, London: Women's Press.
Cobham-Sander, R. (1980) 'Women in Jamaican literature 1900–1950' in C. Boyce-Davis and E. Fido (eds) *Out of the Kumbla. Caribbean Women and Literature*, Trenton NJ: Africa World Press.

Elliot Parris, E. (1986) 'A review of *Minty Alley*' in P. Bruhle (ed.) *C. L. R. James: His Life and Work*, London: Allison & Busby.
Evans, M. (ed.) (1984) *Black Women Writers*, London: Pluto Press.
Gutzmore, C. (ed.) (1986) *Caribbean Women: Labour and Resistance*, catalogue for the Garvey-Rodney Visual History Archive and the Caribbean Visual History Resources Project, Institute of Education, University of London.
Hall, D. (ed.) (1989) 'Above All Others: Phibbah' (The diary of a Westmoreland planter: Conclusion *Jamaica Journal* (Institute of Jamaica)) 22(1): 57–64.
Hemenway, R. (1986) *A Literary Biography of Zora Neale Hurston*, London: Camden Press.
Humm, M. (1991) *Border Traffic. Strategies of Contemporary Women Writers*, Manchester and New York: Manchester University Press.
Hurston, Z. N. (1987) [1934] *Jonah's Gourd Vine*, London: Virago.
Hurston, Z. N. (1990) [1935] *Of Mules and Men. Negro Folktales and Voodoo Practices in the South*, New York: Harper Row.
Hurston, Z. N. (1990) [1938] *Tell My Horse*, New York: Harper Row.
Hurston, Z. N. (1986) *Their Eyes Were Watching God*, London: Virago.
James, L. (ed.) (1968) *The Islands in Between. Essays on West Indian Literature*, London: Oxford University Press.
Marson, U. (1930) Tropic Reveries, Kingston, Jamaica.
Marson, U. (1931) *'At What a Price'*, unpublished playscript, British Library.
Marson, U. (1937a) 'Stonebreakers' in *The Moth and the Star*, Kingston, Jamaica.
Marson, U. (1937b) 'Wanted: writers and publishers', *Public Opinion*, 12 June.
Marson, U. (1938a) Letter to James Weldon Johnson, 1 January, James Weldon Johnson Papers, Beinecke Library, Yale University.
Marson U. (1938b) *Pocomania*, unpublished playscript, Una Marson's papers, The Institute of Jamaica, Kingston.
Mathurin Mair, L. (1975) *The Rebel Woman in the British West Indies During Slavery*, Kingston: African-Caribbean Publications/Institute of Jamaica.
Mathurin Mair, L. (1990) 'Recollections of a journey into a rebel past', in S. Cudjoe (ed.) *Caribbean Women Writers*, Essays from the First International Conference, Massachusetts: Calaloux Publications.
Patterson, O. (1967) *The Sociology of Slavery*, London: McKibbob & Kee.
Rich, A. (1986) 'Blood, bread and poetry, selected prose 1979–1985' *Compulsory Heterosexuality and Lesbian Existence*, London: Virago.
Sander, R. (ed.) (1978) *From Trinidad*, New York: Africana Publishing Company.
Sistren with Ford Smith, H. (1986) *Lionheart Gal*, London: Women's Press.
Walker, A. (1979) *I Love Myself When I Am Laughing*, New York: Feminist Press.

Washington, M. H. (ed.) (1987) 'The darkened eye restored: notes towards a literary history of black women', in *Invented Lives Narratives of Black Women 1860–1960*, London: Virago.
Weldon Johnson, J. (1991) *Black Manhattan*, New York: Da Capo Press.

Chapter 3

Those whom the immigration law has kept apart – let no-one join together: a view on immigration incantation

Deborah Cheney

On 11 July 1596, Queen Elizabeth I issued an open letter to the Lord Mayor of London and Mayors and Sheriffs of other towns, which read:

> Her Majesty understanding that several blackamoors have lately been brought into this realm, of which kind of people there are already too many here . . . her Majesty's pleasure therefore is that those kind of people should be expelled from the land.
>
> (Acts of the Privy Council of England 1596–7, quoted in Fryer 1984)

Repeated efforts to remove Black people were made, the proclamation was reiterated in 1601 in the terms that the Queen was: 'highly discontented to understand the great numbers of negars and Blackamoors which (as she is informed) are crept into this realm' (Proclamation of 1601, quoted in Fryer 1984).

Amidst the struggling British economy of the 1940s, the arrival of the 'Empire Windrush' carrying labour from the West Indies was welcomed by the press with a headline 'Five Hundred Pairs of Willing Hands' (*Daily Worker* 23 June 1948). By 1960 this same population were 'feared as competitive intruders' (Glass and Pollins 1960: 120) and the climate of opinion was rousing the call from politicians for limitation. In 1962 the Commonwealth Immigrants Act became law.

In 1991 a Race Issues Opinion Survey[1] recorded findings that, of a polled 'white' sample of 766, 29 per cent estimated the combined Afro-Caribbean and Asian population of Britain to be more than 10 million; 52 per cent provided an estimate of 5 million. Only 7 per cent of those polled were close to the actual figure of 2.63 million (Office of Population Censuses and Surveys 1991). Provided with a list of groups of potential immigrants, 42 per cent of the same sample thought the law should be changed to make it harder for all those listed to come to Britain.

A 'numbers game' has been played in the public space of the United Kingdom 'immigration arena' for centuries. Vocabulary employed in reporting upon immigration issues is indicative of numbers even if actual numbers themselves are not specified. The collective term for immigrants is in the order of: 'swamp', 'mass', 'wave', 'deluge, 'flood', 'tide' or 'hordes' – the watery metaphors both pre-dating and post-dating the infamous 'rivers of blood' Powell speech of 1968. Precedent suggests that such language is an emotive 'call to arms': the 'Enemy within' speech given by Powell on the eve of the 1970 general election can be regarded as a decisive factor in the shift of public opinion which returned the Conservative Government to power – within a year their government had legislated a new Immigration Act which incorporated the proposals for repatriation which Powell had dramatized so vividly in his rhetoric (see Mercer 1991). By 1979 Dr Shirley Summerskill was drawing attention to the persuasive vocabulary of immigration-speak, remarking of the Prime Minister: 'She successfully fanned the flames of racism and gave the word "swamped" a new meaning in the English language' (Summerskill, *Hansard* Vol. 975, No. 80, Col. 353). More recently the terminology of 'menacing demographic force patterns' (*Daily Telegraph*, 3 December 1991) has had very specific results in respect of the treatment of refugees by the United Kingdom. Comments similar to those of one Minister remarking: 'We can't have all of Africa and Asia coming to London' (Lloyd 1991), have surrounded the introduction of the Asylum and Immigration Appeals Bill in 1992.

Discussion of the subject of immigration within the media is a mirror of the wider economic and sociopolitical debate surrounding immigration. It reveals how unbalanced the 'numbers game' is, in terms of those who engage in 'play' – revealing the spectre that haunts the world of immigration control. It makes evident that when 'numbers' are spoken of that warrant control – it is very specific numbers which are the target. A front page report 'Human tide is pushing world to disaster' is a case in point (*Daily Telegraph* 30 April 1992). Ostensibly reporting upon United

Nations findings in respect of world population trends, the article talks of a 'chilling' report prophesying that 'Unless immediate action is taken to control the spiralling numbers, the very future of humanity is at risk as the planet's resources are swamped' (ibid.). Pinpointing the growth as 'almost entirely in the Third World', the prime consequence is posed as being 'mass migration from the overcrowded and starving poorer countries to the developed nations where growth is under control' (ibid.). This factor then lends itself to inclusion within the debate of how 'EC countries, including Britain, are already under huge pressure from a tide of immigrants from the South attracted by the magnet of their prosperity and stability' (ibid.). All the common currency vocabulary of immigration-speak is present, not least 'Third World' as a term in/of itself which predicates particular communities as inferior to the 'First World' of the West. That these communities are regarded as having tendencies towards the 'invasion' of those 'advanced' areas of the globe upon which survival of the planet depends, poses them as the enemy to be kept out. It is a small step from these assumptions – that they seek the West's 'prosperity' and compete over resources – to regard every overseas applicant as being in search of the 'streets of gold', whatever category of passenger they claim to be; to fuel the debate upon welfare 'scroungers'; to consider every asylum-seeker an 'economic refugee'. The media becomes the accomplice that shuffles the blindfolded targets into the sights of immigration control.

Fears surrounding economic and social conditions are at the heart of the press 'numbers debate'. The personification of all those arriving as 'luxury immigrants' who are a drain on public resources lends itself readily to a case both for discreditation, on the grounds of arrivants being both a 'threat' and a 'problem', and a call for tighter controls (see Van Dijk 1991). In particular the stress on a clamour for British benefits can have disasterous consequences for refugees fleeing for their lives to a safe haven – rendering them 'economic migrants'. The supreme spell of such reporting lies in a bias which directs attention away from the fact that such benefit offices themselves have the potential to operate as a form of immigration control. Matters of sponsorship and maintenance, of ability to accommodate, of tax allowances and benefits, all of which are central criteria to the issue of family members seeking to join relatives in the United Kingdom, provide the links in a chain which bind these and other offices of the state to immigration control and its procedures. Absence of reporting of this perspective silences the complaints of those who fall victim to the extended tentacles of immigration control. Not least it marginalizes the status thrust upon the ethnic minority community resident in the United Kingdom of control – both of their movements and the way they live their lives: the effective prescription of how, even if, they use health and benefit services when the appearance of an applicant can prompt arbitrary checks upon immigration status. Such alienating treatment, discouraging people rightfully entitled to such benefits, is promoted by a press who report 'tides' of overseas visitors taking advantage of the 'liberal' system in the United Kingdom. As one MP remarked in the matter of health authority care: 'The immigrant community in this country may be forgiven for regarding this as yet another extension of internal immigration controls' (Dunwoody 1982). Not only does this provide fuel for attacks on individuals within these communities,[2] it has important and dangerous ramifications. Not least of these is the spectrum of strategic potential it affords the authorities: from legitimation of 'internal controls' as a safeguard to ensure that those seeking benefits etc. are entitled to them, to the 'hue and cry' of repatriation as a force to restrict behaviour.[3]

The tenor of presentation of the matter of immigration and global migration is invariably in terms of notions of 'curbing' and 'restricting' – concepts which have long been part of both immigration rhetoric and practice. There has been little progress from the terminology of earlier centuries, such as that in a letter which appeared in the London Chronicle of 1764, commenting on the then fashionable practice of importing Black servants: 'As they fill the places of so many of our own people . . . It is . . . high time that some remedy be applied . . . by totally prohibiting the importation of any more of them' (*London Chronicle* 1764, quoted in Fryer 1984). By 1772 the son-in-law of the governor of Barbados was petitioning a Member of Parliament for a law designed to exclude Black people, which would, in turn 'preserve the race of Britons from stain and contamination' (Eastwick n.d., quoted in Fryer 1984). Both of these approaches have been more recently manifested. A headline 'House that for Cheek' accompanied a report of a family of Asians who, allegedly 'knowing just one English word – HOUSE . . . repeated it parrot-style as they wandered the streets' until they were given local authority housing (*Daily Star* 24 June 1991). The same paper suggested that their own coverage of how immigrants are entitled to a 'bagful' of benefits 'highlighted just how easy it is for foreigners to fly here and sponge off the state, living rent-free in council houses and grabbing every penny they can in benefits' (*Daily Star* 19 November 1991). The 'stain and contamination' perspective has progressed over the centuries through the rhetoric of eugenics to fears such as those expressed by one MP in the House of Commons in 1979 that:

> Either there are far more here than is admitted, or they are multiplying at double the rate of everyone else. When one localizes these figures, one comes up with the astonishing result that about one-quarter of the births in the whole of Greater London are coloured . . . something like that in a period of only 20 years certainly matters.
>
> (Bell 1979)

Taken to task on why he chose to consider this change in British society in terms of the vocabulary of 'magnitude' and 'cataclysmic', this MP retorted 'there is something genetically different about them. One gets one's genes from one's parents, not one's place of birth' (ibid.).

Such perspectives distort facts, are divorced from the truth, and taint attitudes – so is the legislation itself free from such stain? To what extent is there a point at which this public world of immigration rhetoric permeates other spaces: the private arena where legislation is drafted or the ports and offices where the rules are applied? It is not enough to point complacently to the legitimation of operatives of the rules contained in the litany that: 'Immigration officers will carry out their duties without regard to the race, colour or religion of people seeking to enter the United Kingdom' (HMSO 1990, para 6). The training of these operatives, the institutional culture within which they operate and the sociopolitical imperatives of the government which they serve are equally pertinent to the matter and manner of their operation. The immigration rules are no more a neutral separate entity to be applied, 'out there' and inviolate, than any of the laws of the kingdom, they are equally informed by/informing of, racial and sexual stereotypes. Indeed the very fact that immigration control occupies a space between formality and informality, the public and the private, renders operation of control 'porous' and thus susceptible to reflection of these elements. Sociopolitical forces feed into interactions which form the mechanics of control and thus become the sub-text of the interaction between applicant and operatives. These interactions at ports and overseas posts are structured equally by elements which exist within underlying social relations outside that situation, therefore affecting the discourse itself by reproduction of the dominant power relations of race and gender in society itself.

Immigration law is implemented in such a manner as to be less a fixed and reasonable entity in/of itself than a shifting array of expressions of the law. The rules have unpublished sub-texts, each with their own conceptual frameworks, in appeal precedent cases, unpublished instructions to operatives and the training of those operatives within an institutional culture. The quality of shifting expression of immigration law renders it able to bend with the demands of sociopolitical forces and turn a fixed gaze upon one group, then another, as these forces demand. Primary legislation, embodied in the Immigration Act 1971, is in general terms. The fleshing-out of these terms and the practice to be followed in administration is embodied in the Statement of Changes in Immigration Rules enacted under the primary legislation. These non-statutory provisions which people must qualify under are thus a combination of legal rules and administrative practice, yet are equally protected by the invisible spell that surrounds 'law' *per se*, and renders it inappropriate to regard them other than a fair and equitable system within which all are equal. It is a spell born of the alchemy of a particular rhetoric, a particular group of voices, a specific space. Those who exercise the right to 'define' within this space are by definition the most powerful, and the nature of the power is revealed in categories and conceptual frameworks which are both born of and contribute to the rules. Such frameworks dictate what is regarded as 'knowledge' within the testimony given by those seeking to qualify for entry. This 'knowledge', which stands as 'law', embraces a specific political discourse by seeking to interpret the reality of others. The content and mode of operation of the immigration rules interlocks with systems of domination and consistently recentres 'white' supremacy within very particular 'spaces' of everyday life – 'Whiteness' is the premiss from which others are inscribed upon the immigration plane.

The rhetoric surrounding immigration is as much part of

immigration control in the United Kingdom as the inscribed legislation. There is cause to suggest that prejudices and stereotypes advanced within public debate 'feed into' the way people are seen at the moment of seeking entry, thereby affecting the way they are dealt with. That these popular stereotypes of the 'foreigner' are premised within a focus of colour is not without significant effect.[4] Not least it is an effect that directs scrutiny to one section of travellers – those who are not 'white'. Applicants must of necessity create themselves in the image in which the categories within the rule dictate they are perceived, or fail in their entry application. The perceptions they must meet are born of a 'given' which is a eurocentric model, and the evidence selected for success is governed by this – thus what is 'proven' as a reality is invariably a reality presupposed. Apparent bias against non-'white' applicants goes largely unreported within the mainstream press, a fact which is not surprising given that that same press fuels the notions that all those purposefully seeking entry to the United Kingdom are non-'white' anyway: the self-fulfilling prophecy equation again. It is the rare case that hits the headlines such as 'Airport race storm grows in new case of harassment' which appeared reporting the indignation of a Black American judge detained, interrogated and searched at Heathrow (*Evening Standard*, 6 July 1992). The report focused on the matter as a third case of a Black American (significantly all 'prominently connected') qualified by the reporter as 'allegedly subjected to harassment and intimidation'. Whilst there was passing reference to the fact that 'Heathrow has a bad reputation for its accusatory tactics with black visitors to London' this in no way reflects the enormity of a problem which encompasses such issues as inexplicable rises in refusals of Caribbean visitors[5] or the fact that under the 'primary purpose' legislation discussed later in this chapter 'we have still to hear of an American, Australian or New Zealander who has failed the primary purpose test' (Macdonald and Blake 1991: 260).[6]

At its most basic level, reporting upon immigration is revealing of key issues which are at the very heart of legislation directed towards persons seeking entry to the United Kingdom. The reported rhetoric becomes a 'construct' of the 'knowledge' that is immigration, 'feeding from and feeding into' legislation – selectivity of issues for reporting creating an imbalance which is detrimental to those seeking entry. By consistently reinforcing the importance of, or threat posed to, areas of life which form the core argument for having control at all, the press indirectly reinforces argument for its continuing necessity. This is particularly so given that immigration is consistently invoked as a referent to 'race news' *per se*, which news itself is invariably of a negative nature.[7] A revealing lurid example of linking (and indeed justifying) exclusory immigration practices to sensationalized reporting is seen in the story 'Refugee who stayed to rape' (*Daily Mail* 31 July 1991). This front page headline carried the prominent sub-heading 'It's not a serious crime in my country says jailed man' and carried the usual ingredients of reference to the subject living on welfare benefits (entitlement notwithstanding) and 'concerns surrounding the way asylum seekers are allowed into Britain'. The quantum leap to using the case as justification for tightening control was made by the Vice-Chairman of the Conservative backbench Home Affairs Committee claiming to speak for the public in the remark that:

> The feeling of most people will be that the judge's decision to deport this man was right and that the Home Office was absolutely right in announcing measures to tighten up on bogus refugees. We have to err on the side of caution, instead of being soft with them.

The pivot of the newsworthiness of the case lies in no small part in capitalizing upon the general fears that persons with alien and uncivilized practices might infiltrate the kingdom. In that the West has traditionally pointed towards the sexual mores of a society as the barometer of 'civilization', the perceived chasm between those seeking to enter as refugees and those in the society whom they seek to join is conceptualized in the 'deviant' parallel which forms the sub-heading of this particular account.

Such indirect reinforcement of the belief in the need for stringent control, a consequence of even the most well-meaning reporting, is common. It is largely due to the fact that the parameters of debate in the field of immigration were fixed long ago. Two central issues in this field of reporting, pressure of numbers and economic concerns, were demonstrably expressed as long ago as the sixteenth and eighteenth centuries – to which quotes within this chapter attest. In fact there is rarely deviation from a concentrated repetition of specific key facets in reporting upon immigration, and these reiterate the very foundations upon which immigration control was instituted, built, and continues to justify its existence. Immigration rules are designed and drafted with particular considerations in mind – of paramount concern being such matters as national security and public order, the economic and social conditions of the country. Each area in its turn fosters areas which stand in need of being controlled/protected, in that they are the practical manifestations of the underlying issues to be safeguarded. Thus economic fear as a foundational element of immigration control becomes manifested in categories such as employment; this in turn directs attention to the degree of family unity which can be encouraged without tipping the balance against protection of the local labour force. The protection of the welfare and social conditions of the population attend equally upon this economic category, with the addition of such issues as who is deserving of state benefits and access to the health service. So it goes on – each category of concern being annexed to actual areas of life in the United Kingdom, each in turn being manifested in specific categories of passenger within the immigration rules being accorded differential criteria – with varying degrees of difficulty to be overcome in seeking entry.

Merely by holding the status and mystique of 'law', immigration law is implicitly championed as being 'above' the crude stereotyping seen in media reportage of immigration. Law is legitimized by mechanisms constructed within society and imbibed as part of the social construction of personalities who are part of society – the media fall into quite another category. Yet there is much in the residue of media constructions which also forms part of the legislation. This is so both in the sense of assumptions which underlie the categories chosen for inclusion within the immigration rules and the criteria which must be fulfilled to become that 'category' of applicant, and also those assumptions which underlie the 'image' in which applicants must construct themselves to be successful. The theme of 'nation' is at the core of legislation and an integral part of that theme of nation which underpins immigration control is 'family' (see Cohen 1988). Categories under which persons must qualify for entry encompass hurdles for those whose family patterns deviate from the androcentric and eurocentric 'ideal'. The immigration rules relating to marriage and to children joining a single parent are a case in point. They are areas which attend upon these issues, upon the basic human right to family unity and fears of 'economic migrants'. Each of these legislated categories have criteria whose sub-text embodies a culturally determinist stance upon envisaged applicants. Not least, it is a stance which embodies particular assumptions about women, in that in these areas what 'kind of woman' someone is becomes interlocked with cultural heritage. Further these are areas where perceptions are such as to cause a blurring of focus, the ethnic minority population within the United Kingdom becoming an effective 'outsider within' by virtue of association. Paramount amongst such repercussions is the pathologizing of West Indian and Asian family lifestyles which has serious implications for the way these nationalities are viewed both under the Mental Health Act (see e.g. Cope 1989; Gordon 1983a, 1983b; Littlewood and Lipsedge 1989) and within the Criminal Justice system (see e.g. Alfred 1992; Day *et al.* 1989; Home Office 1992; NACRO 1992).

A strict list of criteria in applications made to Entry Clearance Officers at British posts abroad apply in both cases:

Primary Purpose

It is required of fiancés and fiancées, that:

(a) it is not the primary purpose of the intended marriage to obtain admission to the United Kingdom
(b) there is an intention that the parties to the marriage should live together permanently as husband and wife
(c) the parties to the proposed marriage have met
(d) adequate maintenance and accommodation without recourse to public funds will be available for the applicant until the date of the marriage
(e) (i) there will thereafter be adequate accommodation for the parties and their dependants without recourse to public funds in accommodation of their own or which they occupy themselves
(ii) the parties will thereafter be able to maintain themselves and their dependants adequately without recourse to public funds.

(HMSO 1990, para 47)

It is required of spouses, that:

(a) the marriage was not entered into primarily to obtain admission to the United Kingdom
(b) each of the parties has the intention of living permanently with the other as his or her spouse
(c) the parties of the marriage have met
(d) there will be adequate accommodation for the parties and their dependants without recourse to public funds in accommodation of their own or which they occupy themselves
(e) that the parties will be able to maintain themselves and their dependants adequately without recourse to public funds.

(HMSO 1990, para 50)

Sole Responsibility

The rule governing the admission of unmarried children under 18 joining a mother in the United Kingdom establishes the criteria for successful application as:

> If one parent is settled in the United Kingdom or is on the same occasion admitted for settlement and has had sole responsibility for the child's upbringing;
> or
> if one parent or a relative other than a parent is settled or accepted for settlement in the United Kingdom and there are serious and compelling family or other considerations which make exclusion undesirable – for example, where the other parent is physically or mentally incapable of looking after the child – and suitable arrangements have been made for the child's care.
>
> (HMSO 1990, para 53)

As with so many of the categories within the immigration rules, these two areas make their impact quite unequivocally upon applicants from specific areas of the world.

The 'primary purpose' clause figuring in the legislation has become contentious, indeed infamous, for inflicting upon Asian applicants the burden of proof to prove a negative.[8] Since 1985 it has applied to both sexes whose spouses/fiancé(e)s seek entry to the United Kingdom, and extended to cover women who wish their overseas partners to join them – following argument before the European Court that the rules were sexually discriminatory (see *Adulaziz, Cabales and Balkandali* v *United Kingdom* (1984) 7 EHRR 451).[9] Whilst ostensibly the change in/of itself carries with it implicit equality in departing from a stereotypical stance of women *per se* 'following' husbands to establish a family, the assumption of this traditional pattern is nonetheless maintained by virtue of the perspective upon marriages being less corrected than merely refracted through a culturally determinist stance. That is to say operatives of the immigration rules take a dim view of departures from what is the perceived custom of Asian women joining the households of their husbands when male fiancés or spouses seek to join partners in the United Kingdom. Equally, suspicion has been aroused as to the 'genuiness' of matches, across such diverse grounds as disparities in the age of parties, women being divorced or entering into marriage late in life. Stances of this nature are riven with stereotypical assumptions of 'knowledge' of Asian women. It is a strand of thought which led to the notorious virginity testing of Asian women at Heathrow:

> based on the racist and sexist assumption that Asian women from the subcontinent are always virgins before they get married. . . . This kind of absurd generalisation is based on the same stereotype of the submissive, meek and tradition-bound Asian woman.
>
> (Parmar 1982: 245)

Whilst such invidious practice rightly became subject of debate, censure and prohibition between 1979 and 1981, there has been suggestion such testing did not cease immediately.[10] The stereotype which is at the root still persists.

The 'sole responsibility' criteria was introduced into the immigration rules in 1969 as a measure of exclusion. It was designed to stem the arrival of Pakistani boys coming to join their fathers in the United Kingdom whilst their mothers remained in Pakistan. It continues to operate as a measure of exclusion under the cloak of an apparent philosophy of enabling 'family unity', directing itself particularly towards family and migration patterns of the West Indies. Claimed in 1974 to be 'a monstrous injustice, a rule which apparently applies British standards of morality to a West Indian society which is totally different' (Immigration Appeal Adjudicators quoted in WING 1985: 111), the rule remains today.

Since the applicants in these cases are children seeking to join a parent in the United Kingdom who has invariably travelled here some number of years before, it is impossible to meet the strictest literal interpretation of 'sole responsibility' – a status quite distinct from legal custody. As such the criteria involve proving fine distinctions: whether a mother has delegated or abdicated responsibility for her children; whether she has been a source of financial support; whether there is demonstrable emotional commitment in the mother's interest in, and affection for, the child applicants. A very high standard of proof is required for a relationship in which 'the natural concern of a caring parent for his or her child falls short of the exercise of the "sole responsibility for the child's upbringing" required by the rule' (*R* v *Immigration Appeal Tribunal ex p Sajid Mahmood* [1988] Imm AR 121, QBD per Roch J at 26). The women who seek reunion with their children are thus asked to be 'doubly mother' given their transgression from the norm by their initial separation. The lack of consistency in criteria adopted by Entry Clearance Officers determining such cases (see Commission for Racial Equality 1985) demonstrates the subjectivity of those exacting standards and the assumptions that underlie the categories into which mother and child must fit. These assumptions revolve around what a mother is, what a mother/child relationship is characterized by; what count as 'important decisions' in a child's upbringing – each of these premised in what a 'family' is seen as.

Differences within the Black experience of immigration control are in evidence in the primary purpose and sole responsibility cases which prefigure and reflect experiences of different groups. Equally, the basic differences in conceptualizing what women are seen as are revealed to rest in very particular assumptions rooted in perceptions of culturally specific practices. Afro-Caribbean women are mothers, not wives – the 'breeders' whose family is pathologized. The criticism of the matricentric family simply because it is matriarchal, which is implicit in the Immigration Rules, rests on confusion between 'household' and 'family' (see Littlewood and Lipsedge 1989: 149). Their families are regarded at an even further remove from the 'nuclear ideal' than Asian families – and by default more dysfunctional.[11] The disparity between constructions of ideologies of Black and 'white' domesticity and motherhood have led to a situation where the role of Black women as mothers often goes unrecognized (see Kline

1989). Asian women are premised less as mothers than wives – as 'passive' objects whose actions and behaviour are directed by and ruled by their menfolk; their motherhood less at the forefront of their identity than as part of their 'assigned duty'. The immigration rules which women in both groups face thus embody a series of ideas and engagements with traditional images, which stand as 'law'. Elements of how both groups of women are seen in this regard are a product of the 'naturalization' of myth. These myths are the legacy of colonial slavery and imperialist administration overseas – standing as a historically situated 'legislated identity'.

Medical attitudes to Black women in the fields of abortion and use of Depro-Provera[12] overseas are as much testament to a persistently insidious 'legislated identity' of the 'Black woman' as is their experience of the application of the immigration rules with regard to marriage, children and extended families. Assumptions about family life lead to a pathologizing of the 'normal' Jamaican family where 'it is assumed that a man applying to join his wife in Britain has married her primarily to enable his emigration from Jamaica, because it is believed that Jamaicans do not usually consider marriage to have any particular value' (CARF 1991: 14). Such perceived 'lack of value' attributed to relationships echoes the common currency of pro-slavery writings in the eighteenth and nineteenth centuries.[13] Common to such rhetoric was the interpretation of wide kinship groups as characteristics of disintegrating families and indifferent parentage – a myth underscored by views of Black women as sexually voracious and prone to practices of abortion and infanticide underlying the way they were seen as wives and mothers. The matrifocal legislative approach of the plantocracy, which rendered children 'of their mother's status' at birth, made the maternity of the women inseparable from slavery and thereby denied them the respectability of conventional motherhood. They were 'breeders', not 'mothers'. Such annulment of female slaves as 'women' served the plantocracy in justifying equality of enforced labour and equality of punishment with male slaves. The less immediate consequence of denying them the opportunity to be seen in other than the terms in which their masters had cast them, has been a legislated existence which has traversed the centuries.

Asian women fare no better from historical legacies, being regarded within the spectrum of assessment of marriage motivation as virtually bound hand and foot by traditional practice and ritual – in the face of which they are 'passive victims'. The tenor of the press interest in Asian marriages reflects this focus, premised as it is in concentrating upon a perspective of 'the strange and alien custom' of dowry and caste. This in turn serves to add credence to what was the official legitimation of the introduction of a now infamous immigration rule. The effective ban on male fiancés which was the consequence of the 'primary purpose' clause was presented as a benign act by the government. As the debate in 1979 records, when the Minister was challenged that 'the Government are not the right people to choose whom a girl should marry, and that it is a matter for the girl alone', the Minister responded: 'Many Asian girls in this country would wish to make their own choice. Indeed that may well happen after the change in the rules rather than at the present' (Granville Janner and Whitelaw, *Hansard* Vol. 973, No. 66, Col. 1340). In effect then, it was presented as an action designed to 'protect' young Asian women from the 'horrors' of the arranged marriage system' (see Trivedi 1984). In a climate of press reports voiced in terms of 'Blood Money',[14] 'Caste Out'[15] and 'Star-crossed lovers hanged by fathers',[16] this becomes a self-fulfilling prophecy feeding back to legitimate the legislation.

In such instances conception becomes the 'official knowledge' which shapes 'official discourse'. In the twentieth century this discourse is the matter of the immigration rules – the questions asked of applicants and appellants under the rules; the interpretation of the responses of those who seek to qualify under them. In the same way that cultural traditions are seen today as a site of untenable practices by legislators, women in colonial enclaves were seen as the embodiment of tradition. Thus Asian women were perceived as a site of an amorphous mass of religion, caste and tradition and hence a site for attack and control of values and practices at the core of Indian society. During the nineteenth century the British administration in India directed their attention to practices such as child marriage, infanticide and *sati*. The 'doubly victim' stance that official interpretation forced upon Indian women in the latter instance remains evident today. Official discourse of the Empire regarded the women who sacrificed themselves as widows on the funeral pyres of their husbands either as victims of tradition-bound 'ignorance' (if deemed to be acting out of choice) or as stereotypical passive victims (if deemed to be forced) (see Mani 1987). The polarized polemic of earlier debate is vividly expressed in the art of the time which accorded *sati* the status of either heroic gesture epitomizing classical virtue, or barbaric custom subjecting women into involuntary immolation (see the paintings by Rowlandson 'The Burning System' (1815) and Zoffany 'Sacrifice of an Hindoo Widow on the Funeral Pile of her Husband' (c1780)). This stance, with its underlying assumptions about Indian society, stood as a prominent opinion of *sati*. The equation stands yet, as a pronounced opinion of the system of arranged marriages. It was and is a stance which acquires a fixity of meaning as 'knowledge' from which grows authorized strategy for practices to be redefined as taking 'legal' and 'illegal' forms.

In colonial India the imaginative construct of *sati* was legislated against, rather than the factual phenomena – recorded debate in the area revealing that women themselves were not asked their motives. The perceptions and assumptions of the legislators became constraints which defined what 'truth' and 'knowledge' were, fixed as standards to be adhered to in the legislative process. In a similar fashion there has been a conflation between 'arranged marriages' and 'marriages of convenience' in the drafting of twentieth-century legislation. This is borne out not least by the implicit direction of the required criteria towards arranged marriages *per se* by the perceived loophole for abuse of legislation to be safeguarded against being laid squarely at the door of applicants from the sub-continent. This was recognized by Mr Alex Lyon and was articulated by him when introducing a rule to prevent marriages where the parties had not met. The role was he said: 'not intended to hit a marriage of convenience . . . it is intended to hit the genuine arranged marriage of Asian girls' (Alexander Lyon, *Hansard* Vol. 973, No. 66, Col. 1336). The dangers of this conflation posed by Alex Lyon have been widely manifest, not least in the serious misdirections which the Court of Appeal have found on the part of some immigration appeal adjudicators. One such instance stands as testimony to many in expressing the view that:

> Under the Indian arranged marriage system, an ulterior primary reason for entering into a marriage can exist alongside an intention to make a lasting marriage; this is because such marriages are arranged by the parties' respective families, before the parties to the marriage themselves have had a

> chance to develop any, or any substantial, knowledge of or affection for each other. One such ulterior primary reason could be to gain admission to the United Kingdom.
>
> (*R* v *IAT ex p Arun Kumar* [1985] Imm AR 446)[17]

Whilst William Whitelaw, the then Home Secretary, confidently asserted in reply to Mr Alex Lyon in the above debate: 'Since the rules were changed in 1974, marriages have been contracted with the primary aim of enabling men to come here to work and settle. There can be no doubt about that', there was the repetition of the colonial silencing of voices who 'lived' the reality of what was being legislated against. As one MP put it:

> I cannot accept the suggestion that arranged marriages constitute an abuse. Many immigrant groups have told me . . . if the Government believe that they do represent an abuse . . . it might be a good idea for the Government to talk to them to see what can be done.
>
> (Rees, *Hansard* Vol. 975, No. 80, Col. 274)

In the same way that the evidence of women on the matter of *sati* was disregarded, and in the same manner that the government was suggested to be making an omnipotent judgement, the strategies of immigration control operate within a structure which recognizes a hegemony of knowledges of the mother–child relationship in sole responsibility cases; of husband–wife relationship in primary purpose cases. The evidence of mother and wife are placed below that of the knowledge held by officialdom. Thus the mother's claimed lived experience of having had 'sole responsibility' for her child is rendered mere rhetoric in the face of an official version of what 'sole responsibility' is. Such negation of the reality of others is evident too in the way practices such as customary delegation of responsibility and wide kinship groups – where a sharing of responsibility is the norm – have themselves been stumbling blocks for applicants. In one such instance an adjudicator, in dismissing an appeal interpreted what the appellant's representative termed 'the customary delegation of responsibility by mother to grandmother which is part of the accepted way of life in the West Indies' as an 'abdication', rather than a delegation of responsibility (*Emmanuel* [1972] Imm AR 69). In cases where issue has been taken with such a perspective, additional 'qualifications' are brought to bear to undermine applicants. In one case an adjudicator recorded at an appeal against refusal of an application in Jamaica that he believed of the father's claim to sole responsibility for his child's upbringing that:

> It is quite clear to me that he genuinely believes he has had and continues to have such a responsibility. But such a subjective belief is not sufficient to show a compliance with the rule. There must be some objective evidence of it.
>
> (*Secretary of State* v *Pusey* [1972] Imm AR 240 at 241–2)

Correspondence between the parent and the maternal grandmother, with whom the child resided, was chosen by the adjudicator as such evidence, assessing this in the terms that:

> there is no reason for the maternal grandmother to have maintained this kind of correspondence with Mr Pusey unless she was answerable to him. I regard the correspondence as evidence of a state of affairs in which the grandmother is Mr Pusey's delegate and no more in the upbringing of his daughter.
>
> (ibid.)

When the Secretary of State appealed against the decision of the adjudicator to allow the appeal, the Tribunal reversed the adjudicator's decision and the refusal was allowed to stand.

In operating in such a manner the immigration rules demonstrate that custom can be disposed of unthinkingly by legislators and government ministers. Such a perspective is equally evident in 'primary purpose' cases, where the focus embraced sees 'nothing strange at all in the requirement that the parties to the marriage should have met' (Whitelaw, *Hansard* Vol. 975, No. 80, Col. 255); ignores the undermining of parental responsibility within another culture[18] and marginalizes the family dishonour resultant upon refusal of applications (see Wilson 1978). Nonetheless, custom can, at will, be called upon as an 'authority' to question the credibility of applicants. This creates a 'double indemnity' for applicants, a Catch 22 situation evident in other paradoxical approaches within immigration control. One such instance is found in the way that occasional contact with a parent in the same country by children in sole responsibility cases can be sufficient to demonstrate a responsibility which can devalue or cancel out a sponsor's claimed responsibility, whilst the comparable intermittent contact between sponsor and child (occasioned by distance) invariably detracts from the claim by a sponsoring parent to both responsibility taken and affection held. A 'double indemnity' for applicants operates within the rules at a number of levels; in primary purpose cases for example in the approach taken to custom. Whilst the legal criteria demand that the parties have met (for many applicants this will involve flying in the face of tradition), it is not uncommon for the Home Office to be suspicious of any departure from traditional practice on the part of the applicant. This is particularly so where a woman resident in the United Kingdom calls her husband/fiancé abroad to join her. It is not uncommon in such cases for Entry Clearance Officers to draw adverse conclusions from a perceived departure from Islamic or Pakistani custom, and thereby to suggest that the 'primary purpose' motivation is settlement in the United Kingdom. To quote from one case which is characteristic of many:

> The entry clearance officer was apparently satisfied that this was a genuine traditional arranged marriage. However, he drew attention, as he was entitled to do, to the unusual feature that here the applicant was going to take up residence with his wife and not vice versa. Concerning the applicant's preparedness to do this, the entry clearance officer made the point that it was not because the parties were especially close, or knew each other especially well, nor was the applicant so iconoclastic that he would defy all tradition; indeed his denial of the existence of the tradition damaged his credibility.
>
> (*R* v *IAT ex p Mohammed Khatab* [1989] Imm AR QBD 317 per Henry J.)

The courts have legitimized the logic of finding tradition and instances of departure from it a proper matter for consideration. As one case states:

> It was simply a matter by which the adjudicator was able to test the veracity and consistency of the account given by the appellant. If he himself regarded the tradition as one that would normally bind him, he being respectful of such traditions, the question as to why he was departing from it was clearly a relevant one, simply as a way of testing his motives for adopting a course which involved his coming to this sponsor in England.
>
> (*Naushad Kandiya* v *IAT* and *Aurangzeb Khan* v *IAT* [1990] Imm AR CA 387 per Taylor L. J.)

Despite ostensible claims to neutrality in the role of operatives enshrined within the immigration rules, the decision-making process in the immigration arena is nonetheless encroached upon by a number of assumptions which are internalized as received knowledge. It is not merely a wild assertion that Entry Clearance Officers have made use of an eclectic range of material in assessing the credibility of applicants applying under the primary purpose rule. In 1991 a Runnymede Trust article drew attention to the fact that the subject-matter of a book entitled *Muslims in Britain* was 'frequently being misused by entry clearance officers'. Claims within this publication were being applied as supportive evidence for refusal of applications. In particular the fact that old customs and Islamic traditions were being more strictly observed, as the community in Britain had grown increasingly devout, was being applied to assert that applications which departed from custom were accordingly questionable. As the Runnymede Trust article stated, these points were linked

> with arguments as to where a married couple should live after the marriage ceremony. The tradition is that a woman should go to live in the man's house but in many applications before entry clearance officers the man is applying to join his wife.
>
> (Runnymede Trust 1991: 19–20)

A case in point – where suspicion was aroused in the mind of the Entry Clearance Officer by the fact that the applicant was proposing to take up residence with his wife (notwithstanding that he was satisfied that this was a genuine traditional arranged marriage) raised comment from an adjudicator at appeal that:

> for a Pakistani man of twenty-six to abide by the whims of a girl of seventeen with regard to the important matter of where they would live, even in the context of an arranged marriage can mean only one thing, that it was the appellant's earnest intention to use marriage to the sponsor as a way of entering the United Kingdom.
>
> (*R* v *IAT ex p Mohammed Khatab* [1989] Imm A 313)

There is a bizarre irony in the stance which the legislation permits, indeed facilitates, to being taken by Entry Clearance Officers and adjudicators. In this particular case – where evidence in support of the genuineness of the arranged marriage rested in part upon 'the sponsor's very positive views' – the Queen's Bench Division pointed towards:

> the fact [that] this apparent contradiction in itself raises the question of irrationality in context of this decision . . . if in one context the suggested insubstantial nature of the sponsor's view is being used against him, and in the very next paragraph the accepted strength of those views is apparently also being used against him, he is by that apparent contradiction denied of the right of knowing the reason why he lost the case; was it the strength or the weakness of the sponsor's refusal to live in Pakistan?
>
> (per Henry J.)

Such double jeopardy – evidence arbitrarily rendered applicable to positive or negative assertions on the part of the operatives of the rules – is a characteristic evident not only in specific instances such as these but also in general terms. Thus evident censure for breach of custom (by doubting the credibility of those who departed from it) must be seen in the context of those same officers demanding a break from custom in applying rules which stipulate that the parties to a marriage must have met. This double jeopardy for applicants is effectively perpetuated by a context in which the courts have held stridently that it must be left to Entry Clearance Officers to decide how they do their work, whilst equally asserting that:

> Any attempt to achieve a delicate and detailed analysis of the motives for the marriage is more likely to obfuscate than enlighten. The motives will often, and perhaps usually, be complex and defy such analysis. Detailed analysis also introduces a 'Catch 22' element.
>
> (*R* v *IAT ex p Kumar* [1986] Imm AR 446)

Ethnocentric standards hold sway, as demonstrated in the Home Secretary's justification of an integral element of the 'primary purpose' on the grounds that he could see nothing wrong 'in the way in which our country has worked over generations – that people who wish to get married should actually have met before they decide to do so' (Whitelaw, *Hansard* Vol. 973, No. 66, Col. 1336). It is the very alchemy of the immigration rules that enables them to render people a 'category' and this in turn a 'site' upon which to challenge what sociopolitical forces identify as a threat. Thus for example women effectively become the site of challenge to other patterns of family life. The record of the parliamentary debate in 1979 which accompanied a White Paper setting out the government's proposals for revising the immigration rules in respect of marriage (along with other categories) establishes the sociopolitical force behind the introduction: 'The object of the new rules is to prevent the exploitation of marriage as an instrument of primary immigration' (Whitelaw, *Hansard* Vol. 973, No. 66, Col. 1329). The 'numbers debate' then was central to the government which was looking for ways of excluding entrants who would be a competitive faction for resources, and a compromise between being seen to enable family unity whilst also meeting socioeconomic demands. The wilful use and abuse of custom and tradition is a mechanism of control in the service of these aims, an arbitrary 'supermarket shopping' approach, plundering the cultural specificity of others – a specifically 'colonial' approach. Adjudications take a format which turns 'voices' into 'grammar'; lives into case studies; people into nationalities and women into 'wives' and 'fiancées'. The marriages and parent–child relationships premised in the rules under discussion are surely not only being seen as 'different' but in their very difference seen as a threat – pathologized as deviant by the premiss of the 'ideal' attributes of Western nuclear norm. That the motivation towards marriage in the West is no less devoid of economic, family, educational and status considerations; that a parent may in this country choose self-imposed exile from a child, motivated by economic considerations, is ignored. When subscribed to by the 'foreigner', however, these motives are seen as questionable and thus warranting of intervention and regulation. Word, deed and gender become categories constructed in a political context – that of seeking to stem a source of primary immigration – and these categories embrace roles, within which there is little acknowledgement of a multiplicity of selves. Instead they become categories rooted in an 'ethnic absolutism' (see Mercer 1990) which regards them as part of a culture frozen in time. It is an absolutism in which the media figures by reinforcing the parameters of debate.

So – can there be a remedy to this state of affairs? Can the legislation operate in such a manner as to respect women as distinguished by difference, yet avoid the inherent potential of this approach to embrace myths? Alternatively, can the legislation essentialize womanhood, yet avoid the denial of the specific reality of others? At present there is a fusion of these polarized approaches in that the legislation might ostensibly accept cultural differences in its perception of gender roles and definitions of motherhood, whilst nonetheless operating a dominant ideology of motherhood and marriage against which others are to be measured. The latter element suggests the crucial factor which mitigates against change is who is casting the spell, not the spell itself. The fact remains that the immigration rules are designed to achieve specific sociopolitical ends and will therefore inevitably and perpetually direct themselves towards specific groups that are seen as the 'problem' to be faced in achieving these ends. Increasingly the motivation behind the development and operation of immigration control has been less to distinguish 'what' the problem is than 'who' the 'problem' are. The excursion into the media reportage of immigration within this chapter suggests that this 'who' has been very specifically defined over time. This being the case, changing the 'subject-matter' of immigration control will make few significant inroads into changing the 'manner' of operation. Beneath this manner of operation are long-established strategies of power which construct identities within a variety of political contexts. The 'truth' that the operation of the legislation asserts it strives to find in each case is a 'truth' which has been predefined, long having been integral to the identity of the West. To change the manner of operation would be to invite other 'truths', to transform what counts as 'knowledge'. To do this would be to invite denial of that 'self' which the West has created for itself within an institutional culture which legitimizes both its own culture and the valuation of how people are to be seen and families conceptualized. In the final analysis, it is about struggling to maintain and project identity. The very specific alchemy of the immigration rules of the United Kingdom is to maintain the identity of the kingdom, its people, its practices – at the expense of allowing others the dignity of retaining their own.

ACKNOWLEDGEMENT

Acknowledgement is due to Debjani Chatterjee for the title of this chapter. See Chatterjee (1989).

NOTES

1 National Opinion Polls for the *Independent on Sunday*, in association with the Runnymede Trust. Survey carried out between 23 and 25 June 1991, the sample consisting of 572 Afro-Caribbean people, 479 South Asian, 766 'white': a total of 1817.

2 *Searchlight* (1991) and *Race and Immigration* (1991) record: 'Two children were attacked and an Asian family threatened after sections of the press reported immigrant families had been housed in "millionaire row" developments. The council in question received more than 100 threatening phone calls'. The *Sun* reported: 'Here three months and the council gives them £350,000 house free'; the *Daily Mirror* (19 November) records: 'Racist attacks on a community centre in the belief it had been funded by the taxpayer'. See 'Press Watch', *Race and Immigration* 248 London: Runnymede Trust; 'Attacks follow "racist" articles', *Searchlight* 194: 8.

3 Media coverage of the Muslim Parliament is a case in point – reactions by such papers as the *Sun* are encapsulated in the headline: 'If You Don't Like Us, Get Out' (5 January 1992). See discussion in Richardson 1992.

4 The equation of 'foreign = coloured' in the popular imagination was established to significant effect by this author during a research project investigating the plight of foreign prisoners within the British prison system. Questionnaires sent to the Prison Service staff included the question 'How many foreign prisoners do you have?', and elicited responses such as: 'Total non-white prisoners = 240' and 'We wouldn't normally consider a German as a foreign prisoner'. See Cheney 1993.

5 See for example the brief report in the *Guardian* 31 October 1989, 'Immigration experts inquire into "ban" on West Indians'. Significantly it is a report premised on implicit 'official concern' in the face of the fact: 'The Home Office acknowledges the rise but denies any changes in procedures'.

6 By comparison, in 1990 the numbers refused at New Delhi, Bombay, Dhaka and Islamabad as husbands, wives, fiancés and fiancées on grounds of failing to pass the primary purpose test, totalled 1280.

7 Research which asked readers to recall the type of stories they had read which involved Black people, revealed the highest recall scores in the areas of 'trouble incidents' in the context of race riots, immigration, the Notting Hill carnival, crime and muggings (see Tronya 1981).

8 It is worth noting that the term 'primary purpose' – which can be pivotal to questions asked of applicants, and crucial to the success or failure of an application (e.g. 'Is the primary purpose of this intended marriage to obtain your admission here?') – may present difficulties in translation. One case records 'There has apparently been considerable difficulty in the past about how these words can best be translated into Punjabi, the outcome of that discussion being that the nearest one can get is "the real reason" ' (see *Mohammed Safter* v

Secretary of State for the Home Department [1992] Imm AR 1). Given the intricacies of legal debate that have been devoted to deconstructing/defining/applying this term, in innumerable appeals at all levels, the communication of the essence of the message to applicants is not insignificant consideration.

9 The new immigration rules which establish equal treatment to men and women who marry an overseas spouse were enacted in HC503 on 26 August 1985.

10 Satvinder Singh Juss points to unreported immigration appeal cases of 1976, 1979 and 1983 where it is clear that virginity tests and gynaecological examinations had taken place (Juss 1985). For the debate see House of Commons Official Report 19 February 1979 (5th series) Vol. 963, Cols 213–24, and the Yellowlees Report Home Affairs Committee, Race Relations and Immigration Sub-committee (1980–81).

11 For criticism of the evaluation of the 'Black family' against an image and ideology of a universal norm premised in a 'progressive' 'white' nuclear family, see Carby 1982.

12 Depro-Provera is a contraceptive device. Carby suggests that its use in the Third World is racist experimentation (see Carby 1982).

13 For a particularly invidious example see Edward Long's *History of Jamaica* (1774). The ideas within this became common currency throughout subsequent centuries as demonstrated in Fryer 1984.

14 The *Guardian* 7 August 1991: a report which relates to 11,000 young Indian wives who had committed suicide or been murdered in the past three years because of illegal dowry demands.

15 The *Guardian* 11–12 May 1991: a report which suggests that 'India's racial system is being more strictly enforced in Britain . . . young couples are being harassed and beaten up by their own families . . .'

16 The *Guardian* 2 April 1991: a story from New Delhi of two lower caste youths and an upper caste girl hanged by their fathers who had been goaded by a mob for defying a ban on inter-caste marriages.

17 Dealing with this finding Sir John Donaldson MR stated: 'I am also disturbed at the adjudicator's reference to the Indian arranged marriage system . . . where the applicant belongs to a community in which arranged marriages are the norm, the fact that the marriage concerned is an arranged marriage is of itself without significance. All that an entry clearance officer can legitimately bear in mind is that it is less difficult to achieve an "immigration" marriage under this system than under the Western system, since the personal feelings of the parties to the marriage, and in particular the wife who already has a right of entry, can more easily be set aside or by-passed.'

18 See Surinder Guru, *Struggle and Resistance – Punjabi women in Birmingham*, PhD, 1985, where argument is developed on how the immigration rules undermine the role of Asian fathers in encroaching upon traditional rights to marry daughters to whomsoever they please.

BIBLIOGRAPHY

Alfred, R. (1992) *Black Workers in the Prison Service*, London: Prison Reform Trust.

Bhaba, J., Klug, F. and Shutter, S. (eds) (1985) *Worlds Apart: Women Under Immigration and Nationality Law*, London: Pluto Press.

Black Health Workers and Patients Group (1983) 'Psychiatry and the corporate state', *Race and Class* 25(2): 49–64.

Carby, H. V. (1982) 'White woman listen! Black feminism and the boundaries of sisterhood' in CCCS Race and Politics Group (ed.) *The Empire Strikes Back*, London: Hutchinson, 212–35.

CARF (Campaign Against Racism and Fascism) (1991) 'Caribbean families divided' *CARF* 5: 14.

Chatterjee, D. (1989) 'Primary purpose' in *I Was That Woman*, Somerset: Hippopotamus Press, 21–2.

Cheney, D. (1993) *Into the Dark Tunnel: Foreign Prisoners in the British Prison System*, London: Prison Reform Trust.

Cohen, S. (1988) *A Hard Act to Follow; The Immigration Act 1988*, Manchester: The South Manchester Law Centre and Viraj Mendis Defence Campaign.

Cope, R. (1989) 'The compulsory detention of Afro-Caribbeans under the Mental Health Act', *New Community*, 15(3): 343–56.

CRE (Commission for Racial Equality) (1985) *Immigration Control Procedures: Report of a Formal Investigation*, London: CRE.

Day, M., Hall, T. and Griffiths, C. (1989) *Black People and the Criminal Justice System*, London: Howard League for Penal Reform.

Fryer, P. (ed.) (1984) *Staying Power: The History of Black People in Britain*, London: Pluto Press.

Glass, R. and Pollins, H. (1960) *Newcomers: The West Indians in London*, in P. Fryer (ed.) *Staying Power: The History of Black People in Britain*, London: Pluto Press.

Gordon, P. (1983a) 'Medicine, racism and immigration control', *Critical Social Policy*, 7: 6–20.

Gordon, P. (1983b) 'Mental health and racism', *Race and Immigration* 158: 6–11.

Guru, S. (1985) 'Struggle and Resistance – Punjabi Women in Birmingham', PhD thesis.

HMSO (1990) Statement of Changes in the Immigration Rules, HC 251, London: HMSO.

Home Office (1992) 'Race and criminal justice system', London: HMSO.

Juss, S. S. (1985) 'Administration of Immigration Control in the United Kingdom', PhD thesis, Wolfsen College, Cambridge University.

Kline, M. (1989) 'Race, racism and feminist legal theory', *Harvard Women's Law Journal*, 12: 115–50.

Littlewood, R. and Lipsedge, M. (1989) *Aliens and Alienists: Ethnic Minorities and Psychiatry*, London: Unwin Hyman.

Lloyd, Peter (1991) quoted in *CARF* 6: 7.

Macdonald, I. A. and Blake, N. (1991) *Immigration Law and Practice*, London: Butterworths.
Mani, L. (1987) 'Contentious traditions: the debate on SATI in colonial India', *Cultural Critique*, 7: 119–56.
Mercer, K. P. (1990) 'Black art and the burden of representation', *Third Text*, 10: 61–78.
Mercer, K. P. (1991) 'Powellism, Race and Politics', PhD thesis, Goldsmiths College, University of London.
NACRO (National Association for the Care and Resettlement of Offenders) (1992) Race Issues Advisory Committee, *Race Policies into Action*, London: NACRO.
Parmar, P. (1982) 'Gender race and class: Asian women in resistance', in CCCS Race and Politics Group (ed.) *The Empire Strikes Back*, London: Hutchinson, pp. 236–75.
Richardson, R. (1992) 'Argument and subjugation: media responses to the Muslim parliament', *Race and Immigration* 253: 2–3.
Runnymede Trust (1991) 'Race and immigration', *The Runnymede Bulletin*, 247: 19–20.
Runnymede Trust (1992) 'Race equality and criminal justice', *The Runnymede Bulletin*, 258: 4–5.
Trivedi, P. (1984) 'To deny our fullness: Asian women in the making of history', *Feminist Review*, 17: 37–50.
Tronya, B. (1981) *Public Awareness and the Media: A Study of Reporting on Race*, London: CRE.
van Dijk, T. (1991) *Racism and the Press*, London: Routledge.
Wilson, A. (1978) *Asian Women in Britain*, London: Virago.

Chapter 4

'A mouse in a jungle': the Black Christian woman's experience in the church and society in Britain

Valentina Alexander

The Black woman has many labels pressed upon her, and amongst those most resistant to change is that of religious animal. When she is not Sapphire, the embodiment of sexuality and erotica, she is Jemima; strong, resilient matriarch, eyes lifted exclusively heavenward, carrying her race and all its woes upon her shoulders, bearing them up through her unending prayers, her perpetual song and her faith in the God-man Jesus. This picture of the religious Black woman can, as in most cases of stereotype, only hint at the real experiences of women within the church. It is also the case that very little has actually been written in an effort to challenge these images and to provide representative insights into the lives of Christian Black women. This is most notable in Britain.

In reality, the British Christian Black woman is extremely difficult to generalize about. Just when you feel that you have understood her most essential characteristics a new dimension emerges from the depth of her experiences, necessitating a fresh assessment. Her character has been formed largely as a result of her experiences both inside and outside of the church and, most especially, by the difficulties she has encountered moving in circles where to be Black and a woman carries with it distinct disadvantages.

The women who sailed or flew to Britain from the Caribbean to join husbands and fiancés, or who came to find work, develop skills and build a better life for themselves, all held citizenship to the great Christian mother country. A high percentage of them were Christians themselves, women who had been brought up from babyhood on staunch moral values and Christian ethics. A good many of the churches attended by these women had been established by fervent British missionaries who had worked hard under the influence of the religious revivalism of a century earlier. To the female migrants of the 1950s and 1960s, all of these factors gave rise to the idea that England was a kind of spiritual homeland for them; a place where they would not only find material reward but also, and perhaps most importantly, social ease and a spiritual welcome. Unfortunately, as familiar testimony reveals, these women and their male partners were mistaken. The above considerations, as true as they were, did not prevent Caribbean Christians from experiencing isolation, rejection and racism – both implicit and overt – at the hands of their British brothers and sisters in the faith. For those migrating with the hope of spiritual fulfilment in a Christian homeland, there was to be much cause for disappointment.

The response of the migrants to the hostility of British society followed a course not unlike those scattered seeds in the parable of the sower. In the case of 1950s Britain, most seed fell on hard, unwelcoming ground, and for some this rejection from the churches caused a fatal shaking of the faith and they became discouraged with religion altogether. For others, the roughness of terrain encouraged them to seek new ground in which worship could be carried out in a warm and edifying environment. This journey led to the setting-up of self-organized fellowships, later to become known collectively as the Black Church. For a third group, the cold, hard rock upon which they landed only made them more determined to dig deep and find fertile soil in which to lay down roots. This last group determined to stand their ground and force acceptance through their unyielding presence. In some cases this meant standing by and watching the mass exodus of 'white' members from their inner city churches to the migrant-free, suburban branches. This final group and their children now constitute the community of Black Christians within the traditional British Church today.

By far the majority of Christian migrants from the Caribbean fell into the latter two categories. The ways in which both of these groups have been able to develop and progress within their chosen perimeters has, in many respects, been determined by the contributions of Christian Black women. Although statistics are not available on what percentage of overall church membership Black women Christians compile, it is clear that they form over 65 per cent of the congregation of Black-led Churches and the majority of Black adherents in the traditional British Church. Their roles within and contribution to the churches have been determined by their position as Black women in British society generally. At the same time, however, their relationship within British society has also had a part to play in their interactive life within the church. In this respect, an overview of the historical status of the Black woman in British, and before that, Caribbean society, is of course essential to an understanding of her position within the churches today.

The racism experienced by Caribbean migrants at the hands of the British Churches was by no means their first such encounter. Much of the British-led missionary activity which had brought Christianity to the Caribbean Islands during the nineteenth century had been tainted by stereotypical perceptions of the slave personality. This often meant that there was little to distinguish the unapologetic prejudices of the slave-masters from those of evangelical workers sent out to bring 'good news' to the slaves. In fact, it was their insistence on the thoroughly heathen nature of the slave; his/her laziness, infidelity, dishonesty, lasciviousness etc. that acted as the chief incentive in the processes of conversion (see e.g. Brathwaite 1969; Fryer 1984; Genovese 1976; Raboteau 1980).

Full acceptance and equality was not forthcoming even once conversion had taken place, and partly as a result of this the slaves soon learned that if they were to adopt the new faith they would have to develop a Christian spirituality for themselves that could relate to their own experiences and was not dependent on European acceptance. For some, this meant coming out of the missionary sect groupings and forming churches organized independently under Black leadership; this for example was the case with the Black Baptist denomination which emerged in Jamaica under the leadership of George Liele. For others, this independence could be achieved by appropriating the teachings of the 'white' missionaries to their own experiences, whilst remaining within the church structures. In either case, the result was an independent Black Christian consciousness; a phenomenon that was 'something less and something more than what is generally regarded as Christianity' (Wilmore 1986: 1).

This process of making the Christian message over into one's own image involved the slaves drawing from the memories of their African past in order to recreate them within the confines of their Caribbean present. Conversion experiences were not undergone in a cultural or theological vacuum therefore, but rather were subject to the experiences, both old and new, of the slaves. The precise quantities of African cultural heritage visible amongst populations of Christianized slaves varied according to a range of factors. For example the amount of autonomy permitted the slaves in expression, teaching and preaching of the faith – a matter which altered depending on which missionary group was involved in the conversion – would also determine the extent to which a more Africanized leadership and worship style could develop. Another possible factor (which is deserving of further study) is the extent to which women were permitted to become involved within the leadership structures of the church.[1]

Creolized Christianity continued long after the abolition of slavery. Through the years it revealed itself through a unique combination of self-defined characteristics. These ranged from the presentation of a powerful oratory and preaching style to a sense of depth and experience in the singing of a hymn. It thrived on the heart-felt telling of the testimony and anchored itself on the manifestation of a faith grounded in a face-to-face encounter with a divine deliverer.

In all of this the one overriding characteristic of the emerging faith was that it was in essence a communal one. Its strength was grounded not on individual contemplation and worship but on collective revelation and power and it is in this characteristic that the continued health and vitality of the faith became dependent upon the contributions of the Black woman.

The Black woman's plight during the long and brutal years of slavery has been well documented (see e.g. hooks 1982; Davis 1982; Lerner 1972). We know that through the philosophies constructed during the Enlightenment, she was set up as a deliberate foil to her 'white' counterpart. Through the dictates of a slave economy, she was made, simultaneously, into a beast of burden and breeding vessel. Also, whilst circumstance gave her a certain degree of responsibility over the male in view of her family, she was, nonetheless, given none of the securities and benefits which, in the 'white' world, accompanied such a status. Therefore, emerging out of slavery her position was a somewhat ambiguous one.

In many cases she had, in the guise of mother, grandmother, aunt or sister, been the only one able to keep the family together. As such her role became increasingly centralized and dependency on her unofficial leadership increased. In other areas too, these qualities were utilized and yet leadership did not necessarily equate with headship. In most cases visible power was still reserved for the Black male. The reason for this lay mainly in the fact that once slavery had been abolished, Caribbean society still remained under the burden of cultural domination. In the case of the British Caribbean, this meant that those ruling elites, made up of the 'white' and light-skinned/mixed race classes, followed the value systems of a traditional patriarchal British society. For those who aspired to leadership status, therefore, it was extremely difficult not to be affected by these dominant values in some way. For the Black woman, this meant that something of a dichotomy arose between the role she had developed through the processes of slavery, and the opposition encountered to it brought about by the dominant values of those classes holding power within the society. This headship dilemma was reflected, perhaps most of all, in the situation of women within the church.

From the very moment that slaves began to adopt and subsequently adapt the Christian faith to their own experiences, women played an essential role in each stage of the development. They were there within the forming of separate organized churches in the period leading up to and following emancipation. In the case of Pentecostalism in particular, women played an active role in its character and its rapid spread within the Caribbean. There is, for example, the case of Melvina E. White, described by Roswith Gerloff in her work on the Black Church as 'the most influential evangelist of the early Pentecostal Apostolic mission in Jamaica'. Converted to Pentecostalism in 1919, White was responsible for planting many churches on the island. She also was instrumental in the setting-up of the Jamaica Union of Pentecostal Churches. It is significant to note that whilst her husband, who was also active within the movement, spent much of his time on visits to America in order to align the Jamaican church more closely to its mother branch, Melvina White was more committed to working towards an indiginization of the movement in order for it to meet the needs and experiences of the people in the Caribbean.

By the time Caribbean women began migrating to Britain and practising their faith both inside and outside traditional British church structures, they had already familiarized themselves with the language of resistance, although it had become so much a part of their spiritual lives that it was not necessarily recognized by them as such. Their tactics for resistance had been two-fold: they had implemented a religious life-style which changed an alien faith into their own and then utilized it in the general struggle for the ideological liberation of their people; second, they had created an institution where their specific needs as oppressed women could be met and dealt with in a context largely developed by themselves. All that was left to do on arrival in Britain was to adapt their long-established tactics to a new environment. Exactly how they have set about doing this shall be examined next through profiles of Black Christian women, each of whom have set up for battle within the religious structures available to them in British society.

THE BLACK WOMAN WITHIN THE BLACK-LED CHURCH

For the Christian Black woman arriving in Britain during the periods of post-war migration, her primary struggle was simply one of survival; to find someone who would give you a room, to find a job that paid enough wages for you to live on, to find a face that would actually smile back at you and to locate a church where you could feel accepted and inspired. If you managed to do this successfully then maybe you would have enough energy and spirit left to face the onslaught of racism and disadvantage that faced you and yours in the schoolroom, the housing and unemployment offices, the social services and the mass media. What was obvious from the start was that if you were to survive at all you would have to be anchored in a strong network of support, and it was precisely this kind of life-line that many women discovered in the Black-led Church. Once Black women joined the church in numbers they not only drew from it a strength to help them survive and succeed within a hostile environment but in turn they also gave to it the support, leadership and commitment that it needed to develop and prosper. One individual who well illustrates this symbiotic relationship between the Black-led Church and the Black woman is Esme Lancaster.

Esme first came to Britain as an Anglican some 40 years ago and settled in Birmingham. In her early years here she suffered from severe depression and this was not improved by the lack of acceptance and support she received from her Anglican Church.

Eventually she discovered and moved on to a Black Pentecostal fellowship. She became the church's choir mistress, the leader of the women's and victory leading band, and the school teacher. In short, she found, in their company, the peace of mind that had evaded her since her move to Britain:

> 'I found the joy that I wanted. No problem since then, has overtaken me that I couldn't ride over. Now that settled peace is deep down there. So it doesn't matter what comes along.'
>
> (interview with the author, Dec 1991)

Things, however, did not end there, because having discovered peace of mind for herself, Esme was made even more aware of the struggles of her fellow migrants. Her own healing process within the church had caused her to develop a burden for the healing of her community. This, in turn led to her becoming uneasy with what she regarded as her church's lack of vision for a practical community mission. Consequently, comfortable as she was within the church and thoroughly as she had involved herself in its activities, she decided to move on yet again. The move brought her to the New Testament Church of God in Handsworth, Birmingham. Although the pastor there had, up until then, no expansive social programme, Esme felt that he was open to such a possibility and she, therefore, set about encouraging him and providing practical advice as to how such a programme could be realized. As a result of this leadership a Saturday School and pre-school was started on the premises. Esme herself went on to become involved in establishing an organization to provide care provision for Black women and children. She has also been directly responsible for the fostering of Black children, for care work within hostels and children's homes, and for establishing playgroups to meet the requirements of children in areas with the most need of such facilities. Having already given 15 years of her retirement to the continued struggle in Britain, she now plans to return home to the Caribbean.

There can be little doubt that Esme's motivation and inspiration in this work has come directly from her faith, which in turn has been encouraged by her interaction with the church. Without the communion and spiritual uplift she received from within the church context it would have been difficult for her to have overcome her early depressive years in Britain and live a life that has proved so useful for the Black community in Birmingham.

Nonetheless, what also clearly emerges from her story is the way in which her conviction and faith as a Black woman in British society have always taken precedence over any conventions and regulations that male leadership within the churches have attempted to impose. For as Esme herself argues:

> 'I am a member of the church but I don't work for the church alone, I work for God.'

She is convinced that:

> 'Every church that I'm supposed to be a member of or will be a member of must be the church that goes beyond the four walls and sees the community, you see, because Jesus went out . . .'
>
> (ibid.)

It is this conviction that motivated her to dig up roots once again, from the first Pentecostal church to move to the second even though she had already made such firm ties there.

British society is not used to images of politically conscious, actively campaigning senior Black Christian women, and yet this is precisely the portrait we have in Esme Lancaster. Her work has not been arbitrary or haphazard. She has come to a highly developed understanding of the situation faced by Black people in this country and has gone beyond this to actually commit her life to doing something about it. In response to a 'white' woman who asked her what her inspiration for struggle was, Esme replied:

> 'I imagine myself in this country as a mouse in a jungle, and you are the people who are the leopards, elephants and all the different things, and it's in that jungle I must survive so I have got to watch your teeth, your tail and everything . . . you may not want to fight and you may not want to get up and do something but when you find that you have got to survive then you're gonna do something about it.'
>
> (discussion, Mar 1992)

Esme's spiritual convictions go hand-in-hand with her desire for sociopolitical action. Both are radical and active and in this they go a long way towards confounding stereotypes which suggests that Black faith in Britain is fundamentally other-worldly, and therefore redundant as far as contributions to Black resistance to inequality and injustice is concerned. It is not that the concept of heavenly rewards is unimportant to Esme; rather to the contrary, it acts as her incentive to share with others who may be struggling. As she puts it: 'my bible tells me, freely you receive, freely give, and again it says to whom much is given much is expected' (ibid.).

The extent to which women such as Esme Lancaster have been willing to assert their values within the structures of the Black Church brings us back to the issue of leadership and the somewhat ambiguous role Black women have played in this area. According to the *UK Christian Handbook* (Christian Research 1990) there were some 69,000 Christians, attending 965 congregations of Black-led Churches in the United Kingdom in 1990. These Christians are led by approximately 2000 ministers and 783 of these are women. This means that women lead 39 per cent of the Black Churches in the country. As we will see later, this figure compares well with many of the traditional British denominations. However it should be noted that they represent the overall situation within British Black-led Churches. If individual denominations are examined, many will be found who have relatively few, if any, Black women in positions of leadership on a local and (especially) on a national level. It should also be noted that the figures refer to ministers – these are not necessarily ordained pastors. Moreover, if we consider the fact that women comprise by far the majority of the worshippers in Black Churches, then the figures become, in fact, far less impressive than they may initially appear.

Whilst it may be true that Black women are not represented proportionately amongst the ministerial and executive leadership of their churches, this does not, however, mean that they do not share power with their menfolk in several fundamental ways. It has been partly indicated already that Black women have made substantial contributions to the establishment of the Black Church, and only sometimes has this involved outright headship of any particular congregation. Their influence, rather, has been evident in the structures of the church itself and in areas revolving around the spiritual growth and well-being of the believers. Hence it is most often women who take responsibility for the teaching and organization of children's Sunday schools and nursery classes; women who run the elderly people's day-centres and supplementary schools; women who do the church's paper work and administration, who organize and cater for meetings and conventions. Women are often exhorters and evangelists, they sing in the choir and act as worship leaders. As such they variously set the spiritual pitch for services whilst at the same time encouraging and prompting deeper worship and praise through the manifestation of the Spirit amongst the believers.

Io Smith is one of the 39 per cent of Black women ministers within the Black-led Church. She is fully ordained and as such is able to directly serve her community in East London through the conducting of marriages, baptisms, funerals and so on. Like Esme Lancaster, Pastor Smith found that her faith became most real to her on her arrival in Britain as she battled for peace of mind and happiness in a society that rejected her because she was Black. Like Esme, too, she was to discover that the only place really able to meet her needs was the Black-led Church, and so she moved from her unwelcoming Baptist congregation to become involved in what was then the beginnings of the Black-led Church movement in Britain.

From the start Pastor Smith has considered herself to have a dual calling; the first is to pastorship and the second is to the community. Both are given equal priority and the two compliment each other well, as she is able to illustrate:

> 'I do believe in the gospel of Jesus Christ that it is a gospel for the whole man, and the gospel does address every situation when it comes to humanity. . . . My main function is to provide leadership and to train people and to develop networks to bring Black people together. I must be frank, I want to see the Black race unite across every border; financially, economically, spiritually, you name it.'
>
> (interview with the author, 26 Mar 1992)

Drawing from her own experiences of racism and isolation in Britain and also those of her family and friends, Pastor Smith is able to identify the specific benefits that the Black-led Church was able to offer, not only to discouraged Christians but also to the Caribbean migrant community generally. For those feeling disorientated and alone on their arrival to Britain, the church was able to offer identity and a sense of belonging, so much so that she believes had it not been for the practical and spiritual support of the Black churches 'a lot more of our Black people would be in prisons and mental hospitals, they would be in a worse mess' (ibid.). The harsh memories of her own experiences serve to clarify for Pastor Smith the priorities of her calling today:

> I am involved in the heart of the community. My mission is not just from the pulpit to the pew. I make sure I march alongside the struggle to achieve a plural and just society.
>
> (Smith 1989: 16)

Within this vision, she sees her church, and others like it, playing a central role – even more so in the future than they have done in the past. Her underlying philosophy is involvement through unity, for she strongly believes that if the Black-led Churches are to provide a proper network of support and service for the Black community then they must work together. Pastor Smith's views are significant not only in their practical implications for the life of the Black Church in Britain, but also in the way in which they articulate theological developments within the country. Bishop Patrick Kalilombe of Birmingham's Centre for Black and 'white' Christian Partnership has described liberation theology as being:

> the kind of reflection on the Word of God, which results from and animates an oppressed and marginalized community's commitment to the process of its total liberation as intended by God in Christ . . . done from the viewpoint of the disadvantaged themselves . . .
>
> (Kalilombe nd: 30)

If we are to endorse his definition then it is not difficult to see in Pastor Smith's programme the beginnings of a structured Black theology of liberation for Britain. Such a theology aims to emancipate from oppressive structures both inside and outside of the church. Moreover she has identified a need to include within this theology an analysis of the status of women within the Black-led Churches. By doing so, she ensures that they will not be overlooked or marginalized in an overall struggle for liberation.

Pastor Smith herself is one of eight women pastors of the New Testament Assembly's eighteen congregations in Britain. As a woman she feels that there are specific qualities that she brings to her ministry which her male counterparts are not able to. One of these qualities is the 'tenderness of motherhood' which she is able to incorporate within her pastoral counselling. Another is a level of understanding and care that most frequently comes from a woman's perspective. In displaying such characteristics, she does not, however, regard herself as conforming to female stereotype, but rather as carrying out an important and yet previously underplayed point of theology, and that is to reveal in a practical way the female attributes of God:

> 'God is not only a big brother and a father who defends you but He is that caring mother who touches you and knows how to caress that pain.'
>
> (interview with the author, 1991)

Hence as a woman within a headship role, she is able to combine compassion with leadership and thereby not only to serve the needs of her community better but also to begin to reinterpret definitions of power:

> 'that motherly caring personality as a woman pastor . . . has something powerful about the kind of leadership that one can offer. . . . That's how I see my role because pastoral ministry most times is to do with caring, it's to do with equipping, empowering, building up . . .'
>
> (ibid.)

She is also able to recognize that within the Black-led Church generally, women have taken on essential leadership roles and their contributions to the upkeep of the churches have been so great that were they removed it would not be able to function:

> 'If I want something done quickly and efficiently I put it in the hands of a woman. Women have very, very important roles within the churches, also within the Black-led churches. They are carers, they are succourers, they give. Women are the most ones that pray, that lead worship services. Women are the ones who look after the church itself, domestically, and women do work hard and give a whole lot as well.
>
> (ibid.)

In spite of this, women within the churches have not been given adequate recognition by their male brethren. Io Smith represents a minority of ordained pastors within the Black-led Church. In most cases the churches encourage a theology that rests on a patriarchal interpretation of scripture. Such a theology may base itself on I Corinthians 14 v 34 where women are prohibited to speak in church, or they may be more generalized, as for example, the idea that all 12 of Jesus' disciples were male and headship, therefore, should also be male. Whatever the doctrinal source, theologies, in many cases, prevent women from taking on positions of headship within their organizations and thereby undermine the contributions Black women have made and continue to make within the Black-led Church. The situation is further exacerbated by the partial collusion of women themselves, sometimes through mere apathy, to patriarchal theologies within the churches.

Pastor Smith, who as we have seen has committed herself to both a theology and ministry of liberation, is also concerned that Black women begin to dismantle some of the oppressive forces within themselves. Partly in an effort to achieve this she has established the Christian Woman Help Organisation which aims to meet the needs of women within the community on both an ideological and a practical level. It acts on the basis of self-help; training local women to serve the needs of other women within the community.

> 'Because women are the most marginalized and rejected . . . I thought we ought to have a group of women who are trained to be able to serve in the ministry; not only from the platform as a preacher or from the congregation, but to be able to minister in a social context within our communities.'
>
> (ibid.)

In terms of dismantling a patriarchal theology, Pastor Smith is persistent that a woman's place is wherever God has called her to be. Moreover, in her role as carer and encourager, she is also anxious to bring this point home to the women within her ministry:

> 'I need to encourage women to come out of that sort of slavery mentality, the kitchen mentality. . . . From the beginning, God has never finalized His Divine plan, without including women; from the creation to the incarnation, women have always been included in the Divine plan of God; Eve to Ruth to Esther to Mary, to the cross . . . women were last at the cross and first at the tomb . . . so men are the ones who left women behind but God did not.'
>
> (ibid.)

The ongoing mission of women pastors like Io Smith, therefore, is, in a very practical way, to educate women to challenge the male-centred theologies of their churches. To recognize and celebrate their role as leaders within the financial, educational, administerial, missionary and worship structures of the church and to strive to accept the possibility of their calling to the headship positions within their local and national church bodies.

BLACK WOMEN IN BRITAIN'S TRADITIONAL CHURCHES

Although it is not always possible to obtain exact figures, most of the traditional churches report that by far the majority of their Black worshippers are women (see e.g. Walton *et al.* 1985). The characteristics of Black worship within traditional British congregations, therefore, are very much dictated by Black women. Similarly, the problems brought about through the sometimes racist and sexist structures of the churches are experienced primarily by the Black women who attend.

For some women who found they were rejected and isolated by the British branches of their churches, their loyalty to denominational ties made them stand their ground regardless, or made them perhaps move on to other branches until they discovered one that was less hostile than the one before. They settled into the traditional British Church system, placed their children in the Sunday schools and determined to make a spiritual home within the denominations they had been used to in the Caribbean.

Little research has been carried out into the condition of Black women or their families within the traditional British Churches. From the studies that have been completed what clearly emerges is that the struggle for acceptance has not been an easy one, nor is it by any means over. Difficulties have been encountered on several different fronts. Women have had to deal not merely with unwelcoming congregations and leadership, but also with a style of worship in many cases much more reserved and formalized than the kind they had been used to from the same denominations in their Caribbean homelands. As one Methodist commented:

> 'You go to the Church in the West Indies and you feel full – as if you've received a blessing. Most churches you go to here, you walk in, sit there for an hour and you go home empty.'
>
> (quoted in Walton *et al.* 1985: 28)

This problem is exacerbated by the worship structures within many of the churches which make informal participation difficult and often frowned upon. It is not that Black worshippers have wanted to ape a style more frequently found within the Black-led Churches, to the contrary, as studies such as Walton's *A Tree God Planted* indicate, many older Caribbean-born Christians have been used to a 'High Church' worship style. Where the reserved nature of traditional British worship most acutely effects its Black members, the majority of whom are women, is in the area of contribution and participation. Unable to 'communicate' through the normal spiritual channels, many Black women, even of the younger generations, find themselves isolated within their church 'families'. The racism which first manifested itself in the 1950s and 1960s still affects the way in which Black members of traditional British churches are able to live out their Christian experiences. Rejection is rarely any longer expressed explicitly. However, its intensity has not diminished simply because it has changed its form. In terms of response, it is generally, although not exclusively, through the younger, British-born generation of worshippers that dissent to the second-class status of Black Christians within the traditional churches is expressed.

For example, in a recent study carried out by Kate Coleman she discovered that amongst younger, Black Christian women, 'there was a general feeling of being patronized and tokenized by 'white' Christian leaders. Some felt that they were just making up the numbers. Also they believed that the more Anglicanized the individual the more accepted they were likely to be' (Coleman 1992).

As with an earlier generation, many young women have become discouraged, and have responded to this new racism by leaving the churches altogether. Others, however, have chosen to remain and challenge the different levels of their oppression. Perhaps the greatest vanguard of oppression for Black women has been their absence within leadership structures of the churches. This, of course, has been made even more difficult by the additional burden of sexist theologies backed up by centuries of European patriarchy. This has meant that for the traditional Baptist, Methodist and Anglican churches, the percentage of female leaders is only 3 per cent, 9 per cent and 5 per cent respectively. This, of course, compares very badly with the 39 per cent of female Black-led Church leaders discussed earlier.

The struggle for Black women, weighed down by barriers against their race, gender and occasionally their class, to take up headship positions within the traditional church is quite clearly a daunting one. One woman who has struggled and overcome in spite of the difficulties is Reverend Eve Pitt, an ordained minister of the Church of England in Birmingham.

Eve Pitt was brought up within a Black-led Pentecostal church and became a Christian at about 18 years of age after having gone through what she describes as a 'rebellious stage', which in fact led to her being expelled from the church. This stage was characterized by her becoming disillusioned with what she regarded as the old tyrannical God, a God which caused endless guilt and fear and which, as she puts it 'led to me being even more oppressed than if I was not a Christian'. She wanted to know what God was doing about the poverty of her people around the world, and about those closer to home who, every day, were dying 'with a tremendous sense of unworthiness'. In her quest for the real God she determined 'either to get to know this God more or to tell him to go to hell'.

Having left the Pentecostal church where she felt that she was not given the space to think and be honest with God, she joined up with the Nottingham Black People's Freedom Movement and eventually became a Marxist. However, quickly becoming discouraged with what she found to be corruption and male dominance within the leadership of the Freedom Movement she decided to go back to a church setting and try to work out her dilemmas within a spiritual context. The church she returned to was an Anglican one and although she feels that there are many difficulties involved in being part of an organization which represents one of the great bastions of 'white', male power and control, she has found it a useful base for her own self-development:

> 'The Church of England, like anywhere else, is full of bigots and people who are totally non-Christian, but for all that it was a place where I had a sense of purpose in my faith. . . . I find within the Church of England a sense of freedom. . . . I can go to God with a sense of liberty and confidence.'
>
> (interview with the author, Apr 1992)

Revd Pitt shares the ministry of a medium-sized, predominantly 'white' Anglican Church with a 'white' male minister. She is the only Black woman Reverend in the Anglican Church in

Birmingham and one of only four Anglican Black women ministers nationally. There are, in fact one hundred ordained Black men ministers. Her climb to this position has by no means been an easy one, yet her source of strength throughout has been her confidence in herself, brought about because of her confidence in God:

> '. . . they always ask me how did I manage to be so confident knowing I'd suffered racism and I would say well because I've been given salvation and I believe in my humanity one hundred percent and I make no apologies for that. I think if I hadn't been confident I couldn't have come here . . . because they will just crush you.'
>
> (ibid.)

Having got to where she is, in many ways the struggle is only just beginning. She feels a definite sense of responsibility both to preach out against racism and gender oppression to her nearly all 'white' congregation and also to play a vital role in encouraging the few Black families, not only of the Church but of the community of Bartley Green where she ministers. In terms of the former, she is at pains to express what she has come to understand as the reality of a God of the oppressed. One who does not stand by idly whilst the powerful exploit the vulnerable and the vulnerable suffer. In this respect she makes it quite clear that God is not colour blind and he does care how people treat each other. Whilst maintaining a level of graciousness, she insists on firmly putting across to her congregation what she believes is the message of God's liberation:

> 'It's a matter of saying if we believe in a God who honestly creates a two-tier society; the rich and the poor, the Black and the 'white', that somehow God is going to turn a blind eye to what's happened to groups of people in our society, mainly Black people, I think your idea of God is cranky! You're going to have to think again because that's not the God Alvei come to know. That's not the God we see in the New and Old Testament. . . . We're presented with a Christ who says "I have come that they may have life in its abundance. I have come to set those who are in chains at liberty". . . . The gospel is about addressing what is wrong in our society . . . and what

is wrong in our society are all the issues God is concerned about . . .'

(ibid.)

Her other area of concern and emphasis is in a ministry of encouragement for Black Christian worshipping within a traditional church setting. She has recognized the way in which, under the pressures of the Eurocentric focus of the church, many Christians have felt that in order to become truly accepted as Anglicans they must first become Anglicanized. This has involved the denial of an essential Black spirituality amongst traditional church worshippers. This process is often made even worse by the behaviour of 'white', male ministers who either remain completely unaware of any such spirituality, or who maintain an essentially paternalistic approach towards it. Consequently Revd Pitt finds it necessary to constantly encourage Black Christians to hold on to their spiritual heritage, whether this is achieved through singing and praying in a particular kind of way or by meeting together for the promotion of their collective identity and experiences, as is the case with the Claiming the Inheritance organization or the Young, Gifted and Black group which is organized as part of the Anglican Church's youth activities.

Within this attempt at maintaining a spiritual identity which is distinct from that expressed by 'white' Anglicans, women, once again, have an important role to play. Not only are they more numerous than men and therefore more able to pursue such a goal on a practical level, they are also frequently more intense and emotional in their spiritual expression than their menfolk. They are, as Revd Pitt described, 'more willing to actually look very honestly and openly at themselves' and thereby more able to take whatever measures are necessary to ensure that a cultural heritage is maintained, both inside the church and outside.

On an organizational level too, women tend to be more involved with the structures of the church as Revd Pitt illustrated. They are more frequently represented on Parochial Church councils or take positions as church wardens than do their men. This, she feels, may be reflective of the general position of Black men and women within the secular world where more women tend to hold professional or academic qualifications. Like these women, however, the experiences of Black female members holding office within the church is by no means an easy one as Revd Pitt reflects:

'... they're having a dreadful time. It takes people like me, who are seen to be in positions of authority to go on and encourage them.'

(ibid.)

WOMEN BUILDING BRIDGES

It has generally been the case that Black women have chosen their fields of battle; for some the Black-led Church and for others the traditional British Churches, and they have remained largely segregated within those areas, despite the fact that their goals have been the same. A certain element of mistrust has crept in over the years whereby on the one side there are those women who, having found rejection and disappointment within the traditional church setting, tend to see their sisters who have chosen to remain within it as somehow lacking spiritual depth or completion. On the other side are those women within the traditional church, who may be tempted to view the Black 'pentecostal' woman's experience as over-emotional and legalistic. Although misunderstanding amongst both groups continues to exist, what they have had and still have in common has generally ensured that communication channels, no matter how small, have remained open. Amongst younger women particularly, stereotyped assumptions are less commonplace. There is generally more movement between the churches and across denominational traditions so that whilst church loyalties are maintained they are less defined and exclusive. There are also ways in which women have begun to join together, across denominational lines, in order to attempt to deal with their common experiences of discrimination on the grounds of race, gender and class. These occasions of coming together are used as much to celebrate triumphs as they are to discuss trials, and they are significant in that they represent the beginnings of a formalized and active theology for Black women in Britain.

Clarice Nelson is a young Christian Black woman who attends a Black-led Pentecostal church in Birmingham. She was brought up within a Black church setting, but when she left to attend college she started upon a 'journey of self-knowledge and understanding' that was to lead to her eventually changing churches. The move was from one that she felt was not able to encourage her new vision of political and personal liberation to one which seemed to possess the atmosphere conducive to her growth in this area. As she relates: 'it was at this time that I became aware, not only of the God of love but also of the God of justice'.

This new dimension to her faith led to her eventually taking on the position of Project Development Worker at Birmingham-based Evangelical Christians For Racial Justice (ECRJ). It is an organization originally formed by a group of 'white', male Anglicans in the mid-1970s who were interested in providing a study forum around the area of injustice. Over the years it has changed emphasis from theoretical study to practical action and with Clarice Nelson as its only full-time worker it aims now to challenge racism within the churches and particularly to encourage Black Christians in both the traditional and Black-led Church settings. Since Clarice has taken up her position she has introduced a new dimension to the organization through the development of a Black Christian Women's Group. The purpose in forming such a group was not seen as a detour nor, in any way, as secondary to the main aim of ECRJ, as she explains:

> 'I thought, well, women, we are the Church so if we get women together, by doing that we are not only fighting against racism but we are also looking at other issues where we are being oppressed in the church and that is as women. Because unless the women are free then Black people can't be free because we make up over half the Black race . . .'
>
> (interview with the author, Mar 1992)

The group, thus far, is in relatively early stages of development. The meetings have been attended by Black women of churches ranging from Roman Catholic to Pentecostal, and as well as joining together in worship they have also been able to discuss theological issues such as the status of women in scripture as well as to examine their own position as Christian women in an often oppressive British society. It represents a new and exciting development within the Black female Christian experience, not so much because the women have a forum in which to meet – since this has been a function of many of the churches over the years. It's main contribution has been the way in which it has attempted to forge together the beginnings of a womanist theology through an ecumenical framework.[2]

Womanism, having its foundation in the everyday experiences of ordinary Black women and yet simultaneously revolving around their political struggles for liberation provides an appropriate tool for the group. As Clarice Nelson explains, perhaps a majority of Christian Black women will resist involving themselves in a liberation movement based on feminist models. However, a theology based on practical experiences which by implication have political overtones are much easier to accept and expand upon. Although Clarice represents a new band of young, politically active Christian Black women, she herself understands that response to the women's group and its aims has more to do with experience than age:

> 'I think those of us who have been through the experiences and who are becoming more educated about our history should try and share it with others because I actually see that as part of the good news as well.'
>
> (ibid.)

Awareness of the history of the struggle for liberation is important because it ensures that the women also maintain a global perspective; understanding something of the oppression of their sisters in the Caribbean, Africa and America.

The Black Christian woman's experience in British society has been directed through the Traditional and Black-led Church channels. For the first generation of Caribbean migrants the generally hostile reception received at the hands of British Christians meant that faith was often shaken and in many cases destroyed. Hence for those who maintained allegiance to any church, be it Black or 'white' led, a spirit of determination needed, very much, to be exercised. Resistance, in fact, has been part of Black Christian spirituality from its inception under slavery. This same spirituality has been created from a combination of African experiences and European Christian theology, and the way in which Black Christians in the Caribbean and later in Britain have moulded these traditions to form a faith of their own owes much to the contributions made by Black women.

Later generations of British-born Black women have not been spared the hardships of living life within British society, or, in many cases, within British churches. Not only is racism still a live issue, but they have also had to deal with the ambiguities of their status as women. This, perhaps, has been most profound within the Black-led Churches where Black women are, in many cases, denied full headship positions in spite of the fact that they continue to be essential to the maintenance of the spiritual and material life of the church.

In these respects, the image conjured up by Esme Lancaster of a mouse in a jungle does seem to have some relevance to the experiences of the Christian Black woman in British society. If it is illustrative of her condition, however, it is only partially so, because the Black woman has not been a timid and defenceless victim of her injustices. Women such as Esme Lancaster, Io Smith, Eve Pitts and Clarice Nelson, and the many others beside, have utilized the spirituality that they have partially helped to create, in order to fight against oppressive forces in the various shapes in which they have manifested themselves.

In the process of their spiritual and material survival in the jungle of British oppression these women have, perhaps coincidentally, formed a Christian womanist theology that seeks to assert their dignity and personhood, because they belong to a God whose interaction with the downtrodden of society inevitably must involve the liberation from all sources of their oppression. These growth signs of a structured womanist theology for liberation are both healthy and encouraging, although they do not necessarily come from one homogenous body but operate on different levels. For some women, the structured environment of an ecumenical women's group is the right place to begin to explore and tackle the issues that most affect them. Others may want to remain within the confines of their individual congregations and attempt change through traditional channels; the song, the sermon, the women-dominated auxiliaries.

As the church moves into the twenty-first century, Black women, who have proved so thoroughly in the past that they can exercise a spirituality which is both enduring and inspirational, need to take this faith onto yet a higher level. They need to think about where they are going politically, economically and theologically. There are, of course, many obstacles, but these need not be permanent barriers. Certainly if the faith that carried them through the middle passage and four hundred years of systematic brutality and exploitation is to continue to flourish it will need to be kept firmly aligned with contemporary social issues. Neither can it afford to blind itself to those internal problems of sexism and racism which often appear in the structures of those churches which they attend.

The Black women represented in this study have clearly identified this need and committed themselves to addressing it. Both they and many of their sisters have used the experiences of life in Britain to deepen their spiritual identities and thereby allow them to challenge the injustices they face. The church, whether Black-led or Traditional, is subsequently enhanced by their contributions and able to stand that much firmer because of the pillars of faith and courage that the women themselves have built.

De Church of God she is a lady
De Church of God she is a lady
De Church of God she is a lady
A beautiful lady sat on de hill dat cannot be moved.

(Jamaican spiritual)

NOTES

1 The reality of slaves having an active part to play in the conversion process is, of course, relevant in the experiences of both Protestant and Catholic parts of the Caribbean and also amongst slaves in America. For example we can consider the syncretism of Catholicism and West African religions in Haiti or the formation of a politico-religious consciousness amongst American slaves. See for example Wilmore (1986), Raboteau (1980).

2 My definition of womanist theology hinges on the concept of womanism as outlined by Alice Walker in her book *In Search of Our Mother's Gardens* (1985). Her key concept here is 'traditionally capable, as in "Mama I'm walking to Canada and I'm taking you and a bunch of other slaves with me". Reply; "it wouldn't be the first time" (1985: xi). A Black womanist theology, therefore, is one which captures the historical experience and creative power of the Black woman in the church, as she has sought to preserve herself and those whom she holds dear from the variety of forces geared towards her destruction. In a way it is a means of talking about God that makes Him both relevant and necessary to her existence. This process of resistance and survival is very often an incidental one in that it is frequently unnoticed and uncelebrated even by the women themselves. That it is beginning to be explored by groups such as that started by Clarice is therefore of profound significance.

BIBLIOGRAPHY

Brathwaite, E. (1969) *The Development of Creole Society in Jamaica 1770–1820*, Oxford: Clarendon Press.
Brooks, I. (nd.) *Another Gentleman to the Ministry*, Compeer Press.

Christian Research (1990) *UK Christian Handbook*, London: Christian Research.

Coleman, K. (1992) 'Contemporary Developments in the Roles and Perspectives of Black Women in the Mainstream Churches', unpublished research paper.

Davis, A. (1982) *Women, Race and Class*, London: Women's Press.

Foster, E. (1990) 'Black Women in Black-led Churches: A Study of Black Women's Contribution to the Growth and Development of Black-led Churches in Britain', unpublished M.Phil dissertation, University of Birmingham.

Fryer, P. (1984) *Staying Power*, London: Pluto Press.

Genovese, E. (1976) *Roll Jordan Roll: The Worlds the Slaves Made*, New York: Vintage Books.

Gerloff, R. (1991) 'A Plea for British Black Theologies: the Black Church Movement in Britain in its Transatlantic Cultural and Theoretical Interaction', PhD dissertation, Centre for Black and White Christian Partnership, Birmingham.

Grant, J. (1979) 'Black Theology and the Black Woman' in J. Cone and G. Wilmore (eds) *Theology: A Documentary History 1966–1979*, Maryknoll: Orbis.

Grant, P. and Patel, R. (eds) (1990) 'A Time to Speak – Perspectives of Black Christians in Britain', Racial Justice and the Black Theology Working Group.

hooks, b. (1982) *Ain't I a Woman?*, London: Pluto Press.

Hoover, T. (1979) 'Black Women and the Churches: Triple Jeopardy', in J. Cone and G. Wilmore (eds) *Black Theology: A Documentary History 1966–1979*, Maryknoll: Orbis.

Jackson, A. (1985) *Catching Both Sides of the Wind – Conversations with Five Black Pastors*, London: The British Council of Churches.

Kalilombe, P. (nd.) 'The Black and White Centre and the Development of Black Theology in Britain', The Centre for Black and White Christian Partnership.

Lerner, G. (1972) *Black Women in Black America – a Documentary History*, New York: Vintage Press.

Phoenix, S. (1984) *Willing Hands*, London: The Bible Reading Fellowship.

Raboteau, (1980) *Slave Religion*, Oxford: Oxford University Press.

Smith, I. (1989) *An Ebony Cross: Being a Black Christian in Britain Today*, London: Marshall Pickering.

Walker, A. (1985) *In Search of Our Mother's Gardens*, London: Women's Press.

Walton, H., Ward, R. and Johnson, M. (1985) *A Tree God Planted: Black People in British Methodism*, London: Russell Press.

Wilmore, G. (1986) 'The Religion of the Slave' in *Black Religion and Black Radicalism: An Interpretation of the Religious History of Afro-American People*, Maryknoll: Orbis.

Chapter 5

Naming and identity

Felly Nkweto Simmonds

My paternal grandparents named me Nkweto wa Chilinda. But the name arrived too late. Time had moved on. This was the middle of the twentieth century. The modern age. Modernity had implications for my very identity in colonial central Africa, what is now Zambia.

When I was born, my parents also gave me a name, as they waited for the ancestors to grant me life. This was taking time. Messages and letters took weeks to get to my grandparents' village and back. I had to be called something and my father found an English name for me from a book that he was reading. Nora. In my father's house I'm still called Nora.

In terms of names, I was born at the wrong time. The post-war colonial African society into which I was born was having a crisis of identity. A separation of the old order from the new. Families were literally torn apart, separated by the idea of progress itself. Having an English name was symbolic. It was one way that you could show you were of the modern world . . . could speak English. Many English names were literally invented and appropriated for whatever was the immediate need . . . registering for a job in the mines, registering for school . . . for the future that was beckoning so tantalizingly in the shape of crowded towns, shanty towns, badly paid jobs. . . . The resulting names were fantastic. Any English word could be and *was* used as a name, producing names that exposed the very idea of progress as a sham, a pantomime, a charade – the modern world was a game, you took on a role and a name . . . Cabbage, Spoon, Pelvis, Loveness . . .

But there were some of us who played this game too seriously. We were pawns in a game whose rules we didn't know. Our names symbolized another existence. A God beyond our imagination. A

Christian God... Mary, Joseph, James... Felicitas. At the appointed time I became Felicitas, and joined the world of rosary beads, holy water, saints, a virgin, confession... hell fire and damnation... a very modern world.

I now had three names. This is the order in which they came to me: Nora Nkweto (wa Chilinda) Felicitas. And my father's clan name, Mfula – rain. We are of the rain clan.

Nora Nkweto Felicitas Mfula. My friends call me Felly.

There are many things wrong with the way I was named. The first being that I shouldn't carry a name from my father's family at all. As AbaBemba we are matrilineal. The maternal spirits of the ancestors should be passed onto the child through the given name. This does not imply a female name, but a maternal ancestor, female or male. Names are not gendered. My mother's grandmother delivered me. By ancestral right she should also have named me. That was my first loss, the first confusion in my identity. I was born at a time when AbaBemba men were acquiring authority over their wives and children based on the new ways of the modern world. The right to name me was a loss for my mother and all our foremothers, and a loss for me, who carries my father's people's spirit, I who am denied a continuation of the female line.

However, I carry an important name. Nkweto wa Chilinda. Apparently he was my great-grandfather – and who am I to doubt it, although of course as one who has studied history there is a clash of truths even in the name I carry. The Bemba historian P. B. Mushindo claims to be unable to trace Nkweto wa Chilinda's descendants after he and his wife '... left home, possessions, their high position, subjects, slaves, etc. for love of their child...' (1976: 50). A child that they had only been able to have because of the medical skills of strangers who came into his country: '... the Ng'alang'asa... who had a great knowledge of medicine...' (1976: 49) to whom they had promised the first child born to them.

Ulupangi lwatamfishe Nkweto mu Chilinda, '... a vow drove Nkweto out of Chilinda...'. If he was never heard of again, how come his name lives on?

My grandfather was known as *umwana wa MuSukuma*, '. . . a child of the Sukuma . . .'. The Sukuma live on the shores of Lake Victoria, several thousand miles north of where Chilinda would have been, but easily accessible to traders who came down the Rift Valley, along Lake Tanganyika.

Are the Ng'alang'asa and the Sukuma related in some way?

The name was important enough for my grandfather. In it there is a message for me. Now, as an adult, I find the further I am from home, not just in distance, but also in time, the more I need to reclaim this name, and the position I have in LuBemba history. It is then I recognize that Nkweto wa Chilinda's spirit and I are one – strangers in strange lands – but also guardians of our past.

Chilinda is the verb for one who guards (*ukulinda*), a guardian (*chilinda*).

The second thing wrong with my naming was the very order in which the names came to me. I was Nora first. My family still call me Nora. Also my parents' friends. I can tell how long people have known me (and in what space) by the name they call me. Nkweto as a name stood no chance against progress. My grandmother, my father's mother, was the only one who always called me Nkweto – and sometimes the full name, Nkweto wa Chilinda, when she wanted to make me feel very special. She has a special place in my heart.

At the age of ten, I named myself . . . Felicitas.

Felicitas . . . Felly. There is a whole lot wrong with this name that I still carry as the ultimate symbol of my confused identity. I no longer have a reason to carry it. I'm no longer a Catholic, which was the only reason I took the name in the first place! I had been in my Catholic convent school for a full year before I was baptised. It was a terrible year. I had arrived with names that were not acceptable. Nora Nkweto Mfula. At least Nora was an English name. Nkweto I dropped, completely. It was a shameful name, a pagan name – even a man's name – how could I live with it? And in any case, we were not allowed to use African names – except as surnames – so that we couldn't be confused with 'white' men's children – 'coloureds', as they were called, in the Southern African way. This was, of course, not a realistic fear. We didn't come in contact with 'white' children, in their posh convent in the town, and as for 'coloured' children, 'white' men's children with African women, they were out of sight (out of mind) in special schools, usually in the middle of nowhere, looked after by nuns . . . hiding one of the 'white' man's fears in Africa. Miscegenation.

It wasn't just the fact of not having an appropriate English name that was the problem. It had to be a saint's name. The saint was your guardian, could mediate on your behalf – a short cut to God, or even better still to the Virgin Mary. . . . *She* was amazing . . . The Mother of God. In a society that values motherhood, no one could hold a candle to this woman. She was to be the ultimate Role Model with an in-built contradiction – we couldn't be mothers *and* remain virgins. It was a terrible situation to be in, and encouraged us to dedicate as many rosaries to the Virgin Mary to help us live this contradiction as chastely as possible. We were constantly reminded that our biggest enemy was the desire for men . . . and that it was the men themselves who inevitably, in the end, would lead us into temptation.

I remember with absolute clarity, sitting on the school veranda with two of my friends on the Saturday afternoon, the day before I was baptised, trying to select a name. The book of saints' names also gave a summary of the saint's life and how she/he achieved sainthood.

Saint Laeticia and Saint Felicitas. Saint's Day 6 March (near my birthday, 26 February). Felicitas was the African slave woman to a Roman woman, Laeticia. They both converted to Christianity and were fed to the lions. Actually I don't really know if that *is* how they died, but my imagination has always been fired by the idea of being eaten by a lion, a common threat to naughty children in my grandmother's village. This sounded right. Also there was no other Felicitas in my school, so there wasn't to be much competition for favours from Saint Felicitas. She would be my own special saint. Even at that age I liked the idea that Felicitas was an African.

Felicitas . . . Latin for happiness.

And I was happy. At last my soul had been cleansed of Original

Sin. The only thing between me and eternal life in Heaven was myself . . . temptation, sinning. . . . For the next eight years I tried as best as I could to be good. In the end the modern world defeated me in the shape of Karl Marx (a Dead 'white' Man) and real live men. By then I had shortened my name to Felly . . . (and had forgotten what happens to naughty girls. After all 'white' hunters had as near as possible wiped out all the lions.)

So now I carry a man's name as well. A 'white' name! Simmonds. Apparently there is Dutch blood somewhere on his father's line. The Dutch blood that is so afraid of African blood in Africa.

My National Insurance papers and my driving licence are the only documents as far as I know that carry all my names. Felicitas Nora Nkweto Simmonds.

Often I drop Nora, it is the name I least relate to, unless I'm in Zambia, which is not often these days. I haven't been there since my mother died three years ago. Sometimes I feel that I can't go back. However, these days Nkweto is with me now in a way that I haven't felt before. It could be because of my mother's death. I need to feel close to her spirit, through my own spirit, Nkweto wa Chilinda. Recently I've used it when I write poetry, when I write from my soul, when I'm saying something that touches my very core.

In public, at conferences for example, I insist that my full name appears on my name tag. In a society that cannot accommodate names that come from 'other' cultures, this can be a frustrating exercise. It is no wonder that many Black children will Anglicize their names to avoid playground taunts . . . and much worse. We are still fighting colonialism.

Friends ask me why I don't just drop my non-African names. It would be a good idea, but not a practical one. In reality, my reason has nothing to do with practicality, it has to do with my own identity. For better, for worse, my names locate me in time and space. It gives me a sense of my own history that I not only share specifically with a generation of people in Africa but also with all Africans in the Diaspora.

I belong to a time. The twentieth century. A time of fragmentation, a time of rebirth. I need to understand and know myself from that position. It is the only position I have, wherever I am. In both my private space and my public life. I'm also lucky. Naming myself differently to suit the occasion allows me the space to experience all my subjective realities and identities (we all have many) in a way that does not imply fragmentation, but coherence.

I also know I belong and simultaneously don't belong either to the time or the space I occupy. I carry my history and that of my people. As I experience life, all that I experience is also in readiness for those who come after me, those who will carry my name and my spirit. That is my identity.

Three summers ago, in New York, at an international women's conference, I *really* experienced being an African woman in the Diaspora as I sat with Joselina and Sueli from Brazil. It was hard to accept that these women were strangers to me . . . I was also freaked by the many times women came to talk to me, thinking that they knew me from somewhere. To make sense of this experience I wrote this poem for Sueli, with whom I could only communicate through Joselina.

Coming to America

I am here,
To feed my fragmented self.
I am here,
To see my other self.
When you ask me –
Have I seen you before?
Why do I say
No, this is my first crossing of the Atlantic.
You have seen me before.
I am your sister.
The sister, whose memory three hundred years of separation
cannot wipe out,
Even though you speak Portuguese now.
And I, English . . .
You are my sister,
I know you,
And you know me.
You are the sister that I lost so many centuries ago . . .
But still pined for,
Just to see you
and smile at you,
and, maybe talk to you.

And if lucky,
Hold your hand,
Hold you in my arms,
After all these years.

BIBLIOGRAPHY

Mushindo, P. B. (1976) *A Short History of the Bemba* Lusaka, Zambia: NECZAM.

Part II

Introduction

This section brings together four essays which discuss the interconnections of ethnicity, gender, sexuality and class within areas of contemporary cultural politics. They cover misrepresentations of Black women in Euro-American film, lesbian discourse and inter-textuality through a reading of African-American and Caribbean works, the survival of the Black woman artist within art schools and the relation between African women's lives and their representation in modern African literature.

From its inception the field of cultural studies has attempted to synthesize progressive Western intellectual history, and more recently to embrace a politics of difference – where class, gender, sexuality and ethnicity are 'no problem'. Nevertheless, cultural studies courses and texts often fail to take account of colonialism and post-colonialism, ethnicity and nationhood, with the result that Black women may still be relegated to the sidelines.

Here I aim to suggest what cultural politics, grounded in anti-racism and anti-sexism, internationalism and an understanding of post-colonialism might look like. Alongside the practical, political struggle to which this scholarship attests, is a search for a transformationist paradigm for the future which goes beyond a small-scale separatist 'Black women's space', or the occasional inclusion of some 'Ethnic arts' to including critical race/gender/sexuality theory within wider intellectual debates.

Many Black women writers and artists have consciously set out to construct images which countered what they saw as misrepresentations of themselves and of their experiences, but it is not the aim here to generalize a position for Black female artists, nor for the critics represented here. Theoretically, these critics differ: for while they all recognize the power of diversity and difference and celebrate the work of Black women artists, some tend to prefer essentialist theories of 'race' and ethnicity, while others see identity as something which shifts, moves and is moved at different times and in different spaces.

So this is not a homogenous body of work: there are disagreements and divergencies of opinion among the authors. The purpose of representing this diversity here among Black women is not simply to provide another gloss on cultural plurality, but to encourage debate on the subject of international sisterhood within Black feminist thought and to face, head-on, the different visions that are being explored.

Chapter 6

Creative space?: the experience of Black women in British art schools

Juliette Jarrett

> Every Black woman who survives art college fairy tales and repressive society to make images of her reality, deserves the name artist.
>
> (Johnson 1985)

MAKING A VISIBLE DIFFERENCE

The process of establishing oneself as a practising artist is arduous and treacherous, and few are expected to survive. This is especially true for the Black artist. The artist Rasheed Araeen, who came from Pakistan to London in 1964, was once told by a friend:

> If you want to be a successful artist, stop criticising the establishment. Try to make friends in the art world. This is a very sophisticated society and you must develop sophisticated responses to it. You can't bite the hand that feeds you, particularly when the hand is white and the mouth is black.
>
> (Araeen *et al.* 1986: 123)

This chapter considers what 'sophisticated responses' Black women artists have developed in order to survive their training in British art schools, and considers their position within the British visual arts world over the past decade.

The early 1980s saw a high degree of activity among Black visual and literary artists in Britain. Networks of individuals and groups formed as artists moved to shape and direct their political agenda and cultural discourse. But the mainstream political agenda was changing too.

The Scarman report (Scarman 1982), which followed outbreaks

of unrest in several urban areas, had put a financial windfall in the laps of inner cities. This helped fund a plethora of 'ethnic' projects, programmes and groups. Meanwhile, equal opportunities policies were proliferating across the public sector in a political climate warmed by the successes of the women's liberation movement. Black women, many of whom had been busy in community campaigns and women's organizations, came to greater prominence as the drive for equal opportunities and anti-racism gathered momentum in bodies as diverse as the Greater London Arts Association and the Metropolitan Police.[1] One result was a clutch of funding and resourcing policies that aimed to support Black and minority groups.

For Black artists, one of the more significant projects of this period was the Black Art Gallery, in Finsbury Park, North London, which was the first publicly funded art space dedicated to showing the work of contemporary Black British artists.[2] It opened in 1983 under the direction of the Organisation for Black Arts Advancement and Leisure Activities (OBAALA) and was run by Shakka Dedi, who mainly showed the work of male artists. Black artists were also showing at The Commonwealth Institute, the Africa Centre, and the Westbourne Gallery (shows organized by the Brixton-based organization Creation for Liberation). In 1984 'Into the Open', the first large-scale exhibition of Black artists' work to be shown in a mainstream municipal art space in Britain, was mounted at the Mappin Gallery in Sheffield.

To parallel these developments in visual art were books documenting the Black British experience, such as *The Heart of the Race* (Bryan *et al.* 1985), the first documentary text based on Black women's experiences in Britain. That work paid some attention to Black women's creativity as a means of 're-affirming our culture', 'challenging the norm' and 'the quest for self-knowledge'. The Black woman artist who, during this period, did the most to enable others to show their work was Lubaina Himid. She curated 'The Thin Black Line', the first group exhibition of Black women artists, at the Institute of Contemporary Arts in London, and ran her own gallery, The Elbow Room, at London Bridge.

Black artists were certainly gaining ground, but there were contra-indications. The terms on which their work was being promoted were far from satisfactory. For example, 'The Thin Black Line' was not in the main gallery of the ICA and the curator was consequently paid a paltry £250 for her six months' work. But political pressures were at work: 'The Greater London Council had threatened to withdraw its considerable contribution to the ICA if something black did not appear that financial year', Himid has recorded (Himid 1992: 65).

However, in spite of the boost to the Black arts sector during the 1980s, there are still only a small number of mainstream galleries involved in organizing group and solo exhibitions of Black women artists' work. Major galleries such as the Hayward ('The Other Story', 1989), Cornerhouse ('The Image Employed', 1987) and the Whitechapel ('From Two Worlds', 1986) provided one-off mixed shows only after persistent pressure, while regional galleries such as Rochdale Museum and Art Gallery, the Ikon Art Gallery and Walsall Museum and Art Gallery have a more consistent approach to bringing the work of Black artists into the critical public domain. The artist Marlene Smith, curator of the Black Art Gallery in North London in the early 1990s believes that the promotion of Black artists is so random because it is left to the personal choice of individual curators and not systematic decision-making. She also notes with alarm that since the intense exhibition activities of the 1980s the number of Black women artists showing work has declined. A number of reasons can be cited for this. Many have given up their studio space, having lost financial support from funding bodies during the economic recession. Some are simply exhausted after a decade of relatively vigorous activity during which they were their own agents, exhibition organizers, reviewers and publishers (ibid.).

But it would be a mistake to give the impression that there were many exhibitions by Black women during the 1980s. From 1980 to 1990 there were only eight solo exhibitions by Black women in mainstream galleries. And work goes on.

THE 'COLOUR' IN CULTURE

> ... whoever cannot tell himself the truth about his past is trapped in it, is immobilised in the prison of his undiscovered self.
>
> (Baldwin 1985: 318)

Marcus Garvey, the early twentieth-century Black nationalist leader, sought, through his Pan Africanist Movement, to unite peoples of the African Diaspora by recognizing their shared roots and experience. Then, the object was the struggle for freedom from colonization and imperialism. Now the struggle is against racism and inequality and for a distinct cultural integrity. For Black minorities in communities as diverse as West Germany, the United Kingdom and the United States, Garveyism is still relevant.

At art school, this struggle for cultural integrity is often acute, and acutely felt. Here, to continue the advice given to Araeen, a 'sophisticated response' would mean to be 'other' than oneself to gain acceptance. But this might be at the cost of losing touch with one's own reality, with potentially profound consequences for the art student. The alternative – affirming one's 'Blackness' against the dominant 'white' culture – results in a state of constant tension, manifested in the often reactive nature of Black culture, particularly in the drive to counter negative imagery.

The Black woman at art school frequently finds herself in conflict with the *status quo* – acceptance or rejection of which will mean the difference between success and failure. Some of us choose to work quietly, wishing not to draw any particular attention to our presence; others will make demands and challenge the tutors and what they represent. But we are so few in numbers that our presence, regardless of how we might choose to present ourselves, will attract attention and even be perceived as a threat to the established order.

> 'At first I found the staff there to be quite apprehensive about what they should be doing with me . . . I found it quite frightening to be there at first. . . . Certain members of staff just steered clear of me, probably because they didn't know if I wanted to be treated differently because I was Black, or just because I was there . . .'
>
> (interview with the author, June 1988)

A large part of the established order at art school is the history of, and devotion to, Western high art. For 'white' women, this holds the image of Madonna and child, and the idea of the female ('white') body 'for the desiring masculine gaze' which is at the heart of high art visual representation, exemplified by artists such as Titian, Rubens and Ingres. For Black women there is the Black 'mammy', idealized for her ability to nurture 'white' babies, rather than her own. Or the contradictory images of Black woman's sexual promiscuousness, and, again, as asexual beings. Manet's

Olympia, with the Black servant in the background is just one of many (Garb 1986). When a Black women enters art school, preconceived notions about who she is, why she is there and how she will cope, frequently manifest themselves. 'White' women may view her as 'strong', but think of her as weak in her dealings with men. Staff may assume that she comes from an oppressive family that wants to tie her to a burdensome domestic existence, and regard her presence in art school as an act of rebellion. While the 'white' men may view her as problematic and 'unfeminine'; they may be troubled as to her reasons for coming to art school. As one hostile tutor said to me, 'It has nothing to do with you.'

ART SCHOOLS AND CULTURAL HEGEMONY

The art critic Richard Cork has likened many contemporary artists to 'laboratory researchers', absorbed in highly specialized experimentation. He cites the influential critic and painter Roger Fry, who believed art should stand outside the 'vulgar social world', serving its own purposes and pursuing its own goals (Fry, 1978).

Generations of radical artists have rejected the principle of 'art for art's sake', but for Black artists the challenge has particular urgency. Keith Piper, who has actively promoted a politically informed discourse on Black art, sees no relevance in Fry's attitude for the Black art student because 'his very "Blackness" is at the core of "social tension" ' (Piper 1981). Kwesi Owusu, the African film maker and writer has argued, in relation to Black writers, that the main reason for the exclusion of innovative Black artists is the notion that 'art pursues purposes and states above the domains of ideology and politics' (Owusu 1986: 122).

There is not, of course, one simplified philosophy within the Black artistic community in Britain. The 'Image Employed' exhibition curated by Keith Piper in 1987 aimed to show the diversity of innovation among Black artists as well as commonality of purpose. The exhibition, which sought to advance a critical context for the work, demonstrated that the artists were as interested in form as in content and context.

Ironically, however, Western high art may owe its survival to its ability to incorporate the energy of vigour of those working on its margins. Black and Third World 'political and cultural

street artists' challenge the canon – or society – but are then accommodated within it.

But, to complicate the politics of art, must be added the politics of being the artist. While the artist has, historically, been constructed as male, independent, anti-social and having a creative prerogative, the 'woman artist' struggles with the view, according to the Marxist feminist critic Griselda Pollock, that her work is 'social', feminine and therefore not real art – which is masculine.

A Black woman artist, however, cannot be perceived solely within the 'feminine' stereotype. Racist definitions, meanings and identities prescribe a specific political agenda for her, whether she chooses to become fully engaged with it or not. Thus art school becomes a site for the reproduction of social and political relations (sexism, racism, and the culture of class) as well as for the production of 'universalization of meaning'.

A Black woman in art school may cause consternation because she symbolizes cultural as well as sexual opposition. Furthermore, as her womanhood is defined and imaged by the 'white' male as subordinate to 'white' female, she can be seen as subversive of established hierarchies in which 'white' women are, themselves, inescapably implicated.

Black feminist theorists such as Hazel Carby and bell hooks have discussed in detail the relation between much feminist discourse and Black women's lives (see e.g. Carby 1987; Smith 1986; Davis 1982; hooks 1989; Riley 1985; Sulter 1990). Radical feminist theory, they argue, cannot adequately analyse the complex relations in Black communities, and fails to acknowledge its class base. The notion of 'universal patriarchy' is often seen as a form of theoretical imperialism that ignores the specific environment which produced it and fails to take account of Black men's relative lack of power in relation to 'white' men. Racist ideology has, in other words, been instrumental in shaping Black men's relationship with Black women, the Black community, and 'white' society.

Black feminism has also argued that Black women have never had the privilege of protection from 'white' male power, while 'white' women have enjoyed such protection from Black men. Thus a concept of universal patriarchy helps to perpetuate a racist mythology about the threat of Black men to 'white' female sexuality, as Angela Davis's critique of Susan Brownmiller showed (Davis 1981).

In art school control is almost universally in the hands of 'white' men. Moreover Black women frequently find that their 'white' sisters behave as oppressively as their male colleagues and tutors:

> '... I found sometimes that they were quite inquisitive as to what I was doing all the time besides work. I don't know whether it did affect the way I was assessed but they were always asking what I did, as though because I am a Black woman I must go out and do different things compared to other women ...'
>
> (interview with the author, June 1988)

Indeed, Black women are sometimes driven to seek the protection of ('white') male tutors:

> '... She [a 'white' woman tutor] still wouldn't do anything, she wouldn't change it even though I could prove to her that she was wrong. I had actually to go to the head tutor to get him to talk to her. He actually dragged her out to apologize to me for giving me the wrong mark – and she apologized to him. I was standing right in front of her and she apologized to him ...'
>
> (ibid.)

Race and sex oppression are inseparable historical experiences for us; for a Black woman in art school, resisting subordination and manipulation is not simply a matter of fighting male privilege or having a feminist consciousness.

It seems likely that the problems which Black women face in art schools reflect the experiences of other Black women in higher education. Little published material exists for the British situation, though bell hooks, the African-American writer, has described her own experience:

> We were terrorized. As an undergraduate, I carefully avoided those professors who made it clear that the presence of any Black students in their classes was not desired.... They did not make direct racist statements. Instead, they communicated their message in subtle ways – forgetting to call your name when reading the roll, avoiding looking at you, pretending they do not hear you when you speak, and at times ignoring you altogether.
>
> (hooks 1989: 56–7)

In the absence of similar autobiographical accounts for Britain, it is useful to note Sally Tomlinson's work on Black women's experiences. She placed their individual achievements within a broader theoretical framework of pupil aspirations and demands made on the education system (Tomlinson 1984). Tomlinson also highlighted students' concerns regarding low teacher expectations, lack of sensitivity for (Black) cultural inheritance and the significance of parental intervention and vigilance. My own research showed that parents played an important role in giving support to the women's aspirations and did not hinder their desire to study at art school:

> '[My mum] . . . doesn't understand fully why I am doing what I am doing, she just knows that I am doing it because I enjoy it, and that's fine, no questions – no nothing, just do it'.
>
> (quoted in Jarrett 1989)

And the women in my sample all had very positive things to say about their school experience. The schools had offered them a wide range of curriculum options and they felt they had been given encouragement from their teachers:

> 'I knew what I wanted to do at an early age. While I was at school I was always interested in art. My lecturers/teachers, they did push me. I took one of my O-levels a year earlier, that was how much they wanted to push me. I passed that and then attended an all-girls school in North London.'
>
> (interview with the author 1988)

Another woman explained:

> 'It was just a normal secondary school. I decided to stay on for an extra year, because I couldn't decide what to do . . . they always wanted the best for you: when I say that they still didn't catch that I was dyslexic . . . they didn't find out until I was 17/18 [years old] . . . I still left with seven O-levels . . .'
>
> (ibid.)

Such comments illustrate how Black students' confidence in their ability to achieve academic success can be enhanced by the teachers taking an active and positive interest in the students' academic well-being. The women's attitude to school and their successes there seem to support the findings of a number of studies which have been done on Black girls in secondary education (Driver 1980; Fuller 1980; Riley 1985). Their success at school is a result of demands on the school system to recognize their abilities; why should the art school system not perform as well?

The absence of equal opportunities and multi-cultural education policies may account for the difference. For the Black girls who needed this politically informed education, the transition from secondary school to art school was retrogressive:

> 'While I was at school there was a lot of changes going on. They were introducing Urdu as an 'O' level subject and an 'A' level subject.... There wasn't a lot being said – not a lot I heard of – in the art school context. We were encouraged to look at artists from every walk of life, but nothing more than that.'
>
> (ibid.)

Another woman explained to me:

> 'I was actually on the academic board meeting. They kept postponing Gavin Jantjes's[3] [visit] who was to speak to us about a multi-cultural college. We're slap bang on the Peckham High Road and there were hardly any Black people at that college, and it didn't reflect the actual environment. He just kept being put off... it never happened – it didn't seem important. The tutors on the board felt that they had nothing to answer to at all; they were OK, they didn't need anyone else giving them more guidelines on how to handle anything.'
>
> (ibid.)

AN AUTOBIOGRAPHICAL STATEMENT

As a parent of an 18-year-old Black boy, who is, at the time of writing, in his last year of A-levels at school, I feel more acutely aware than my parents were that my knowledge of the traps, obstacles and shortcomings of the education system, when dealing (encouragingly) with Black pupils, boys in particular, will contribute to his academic achievements. Casual stereotyping of both my son as a potential non-achiever and agent of potential disruption, and the branding of me as a parent with too high expectations and inadequate understanding of how children learn are obstacles a majority of Black parents have had to face. My son's father and I have had to engage in serious fisticuffs with both school and local education authority over a mostly fictional assessment of his character and ability.

One of my responsibilities as a Black parent is to anchor my son in a cultural identity with its roots stretching back to Africa via the Caribbean. We, his parents, are the products of the intellectually demanding Black liberation movement of the 1960s and 1970s. We emerged from that period with strong political views on Black achievement past, present and future. Our generation's thirst for knowledge and information encouraged by our young aunts and uncles and parents gave rise to the concept of Black culture as a shorthand for cultural resistance.

I take the view that 'Black' is a political statement, 'Black culture' is a historical imperative, and the 'Black artist' is a cultural necessity; so whether one is politically motivated or not, one will be forced to take a political stance in dealing with the representatives of 'white' male hegemony. Black artists must find means to make their work visible in the public domain. But, public exposure will not be enough; we will need to continue to develop a body of published critical texts that discusses the artist, the work itself and the issues surrounding it.

Unlike the women in my sample who were, on average, 12 years younger than me, I entered art school having experienced the rejuvenating effects, as a teenager, of the Black power movement of the 1970s. It had filled me with a sense of self-worth and had encouraged in me a determination to value learning, both self-pursued and state provided, but not to accept it unquestioningly. It had also provided me with a voice that knew how to phrase a demand for knowledge which would acknowledge my history more honestly. Paradoxically, just as art school had fanned the cult of the artist as individual/loner, I learnt how to draw on my own resources, exposed as I often was to being the 'lone' Black in institutional settings.

My wish in art school was to learn about Western art and its influences and Black art and its developments. But art school seemed unable to offer this without making me feel alienated from the real purpose of the place, which was to promote high art culture. In responding to my demands in that manner, it enabled my tutors to view me as problematic, allowing those who should be held accountable to sidestep their responsibility. My tutors were of little use to me when I was formulating my research outline on the 'Black Tradition in Western Art' for my final year dissertation. Even if my demands for a particular type of knowledge that reflected my past and present contribution had been satisfied I would still have been concerned about the way the knowledge could be presented without becoming debased and marginalized. However, had such knowledge been offered I would have taken it up and made it my own. The women I interviewed had similar needs and aspirations, and their tutors' response to their work and their desire to make contact with other Black artists was, again, similar.

Stress is placed on the validation of work through the gallery system in art school; but Black artists are generally considered to be on the periphery of mainstream art activity. Art school neither promotes Black art nor encourages Black students to explore those exhibition venues where they could locate Black artists who might share with them similar ethical and aesthetic values. Consequently, Black art students are denied the opportunity to make a crucial link between the perception of themselves as isolated Black artists and identification with a body of critical discourse on Black art and creativity.

Black art students are left to find relevant galleries, resources and artists on their own. Within the Black art movement, they may find that what is demanded of them, in terms of context and content, may be diametrically opposed to that which is promoted as acceptable in art school.

It is difficult to resist the pressure to conform to the predominant ethos of the art school environment, particularly when a refusal to do so could leave one further isolated by the mainstream:

> 'I'm very independent. I think I am a stubborn person – I wouldn't like to change myself to suit someone . . . I really respect those who are proud of their culture, and it shows in them – everything comes out – that's what I expect Black artists to be doing: portraying your own culture.'
>
> (ibid.)

Although many of the young Black women were not politically active in the usual sense, they resisted others' attempts to define their identity, even to the extent that their behaviour might be interpreted as a denial of 'Blackness':

> 'There was one lecturer who said, because I became interested in textiles when I was on my foundation course, 'Why don't you read some books on African art, you might like that?' I just ignored him, and walked away.
>
> 'I remember I had, not an argument as such, but a discussion with one of the 'white' students at college who was middle class and she knew what life was about. She kept saying that I wanted to be middle class; I had gone to art college therefore I must be aspiring to something else; I must be denying what I am to gain something else. She couldn't accept it was what I wanted to do – because Black people, Black women didn't do that; I had to want to be something else.'
>
> (ibid.)

But often the greatest problem faced by many Black women in art schools, as in other areas of higher education, is isolation. As solitary people, each woman knows she must assert herself and express her point of view to survive. Yet that same freedom of expression may jeopardize her sense of security and make her more vulnerable. It is always a question of maintaining a delicate balance.

> 'In a way I've actually started living now, actually finding out what's out there. I need to become acquainted with all that. The problem now is actually finding out where everything is, that is the real problem. Just not being aware of anything, I didn't realize how isolated I was.'
>
> (ibid.)

Another woman explained:

> 'I think right from the beginning of the course I made my points clear to the college or to the head of the department, that I wasn't prepared to change my style. I'm just coming to learn what I can from here and that's about it really and no one has the right to criticize what I do or not. If I need help, I ask for it, if I don't – just forget it . . .'
>
> (ibid.)

The contradictions which students face if they cut themselves off from the whole group, or remain silent in the face of arrogant assertions about their work, preferring to trust their own counsel, are clear.

Although Black women in art schools may feel they lose something of their cultural heritage in order to survive, they also recognize the need to network with the 'white' women in spite of the risks:

> 'Sometimes you just didn't want to talk to a tutor because they were sometimes just not the right person to see at that time, you need someone you can trust to look at your work . . . all the women stuck together because we knew we could do it. We were just as good as the men – we were together on that.

> 'When I was at art school I do not believe that the art establishment had any particular expectation about what type of art I should produce beyond paying homage to the 'great masters'. It was understood that Black artists had contributed nothing to the way things were viewed – it was not considered to be my inherited aesthetic territory; the influence of African art on Western art traditions had escaped rational recognition. The assumption was, therefore, that I would emulate the European, like any other student would have done. There was, however, self-imposed pressure to produce a politically viable and culturally specific art.
>
> (ibid.)

But in the absence of contact with practising Black artists, this is very difficult to achieve. Few tutors routinely network with Black artists and so are unable to refer students to 'works' or exhibition locations. As a result, few of the women I interviewed were familiar with Black art groups or individuals' work; they had to take the initiative if they wanted to engage in the critical discourse on Black art and locate their work in a broader creative context:

> 'While I was at art school I contacted the Black Art Gallery . . . [it] deals with works which show the experience of Black people within the society rather than what Black artists are doing . . . I think that my work is still valid as a Black artist even though it's not experiences of Black people . . . but to me it's the experience of a Black artist's work which is also

important. . . . It is an important part that I am a Black woman who is also an artist . . . I don't think it should be ignored.'

(ibid.)

In response to her own question, 'What did it mean for a Black woman to be an artist in our grandmothers' time? In our great-grandmothers' day?', Alice Walker replied, the answer was 'cruel enough to stop the blood'. Even today, the task of learning to be an artist is for many Black women a battle, but one worth fighting:

'I've found it probably one of the most difficult experiences. Maybe it's because of the choice of college I made. I don't know whether it would have been different if I'd gone somewhere in central London. I think it would probably have been quite different, but I don't know. I found it a really hard experience, but I'm glad I've gone through it 'cos I've learnt loads of things about myself and I think my character has changed and developed and got stronger because of it.'

(ibid.)

Some feel strong enough to go back for more:

'I am hoping to do postgrad.'

NOTES

1 The Greater London Council (GLC) and later the Inner London Education Authority (ILEA) took a strong lead in the development of equal opportunities policies that had an avowed aim to benefit those sections of society that were identified as disadvantaged. The principles underlying the ILEA texts for equality, published in a series of policy documents entitled Race, Sex and Class, were widely adopted by bodies such as the Arts Council, the Greater London Arts Association, the Calouste Gulbenkian Foundation, the Community Relations Executive, even the defunct Manpower Services Commission. Financial support was given to minority arts groups, and the Minority Arts Advisory Service, a funded body, helped to co-ordinate the sector.
2 This gallery closed in 1993 due to lack of funding.
3 Gavin Jantjes is a Black South African painter and has been Senior Lecturer at the London Institute since 1986.

BIBLIOGRAPHY

Araeen, R., Kirby, R. and Serota, N. (1986) *From Two Worlds*, London: Trustees of the Whitechapel Art Gallery.

Baldwin, J. (1985) *The Price of the Ticket*, London: Michael Joseph.

Bryan, B., Dadzie, S. and Scafe, S. (1985) *Heart of the Race*, London: Virago.

Carby, H. (1987) *Reconstructing Womanhood: The Emergence of the Afro-American Woman Novelist*, Oxford: Oxford University Press.

Davis, A. (1982) *Women, Race and Class*, London: The Women's Press.

Driver, G. (1980) 'How West Indians do better at school – (especially the girls)' *New Society*, 17 January.

Fry, R. (1978) *Art for Whom?*, London: Arts Council of Great Britain.

Fuller, M. (1980) 'Black girls in a London comprehensive school' in R. Deen (ed.) *Schooling for Women's Work*, London: Routledge & Kegan Paul.

Garb, T. (1986) 'Art, History, Race', lecture given at the University of London, Institute of Education, December.

Himid, L. (1992) 'Mapping: a decade of Black women artists 1980–1990' in M. Sulter (ed.) *Passion: Discourses on Black Women's Creativity*, Hebden Bridge: Urban Fox Press.

hooks, b. (ed.) (1989) 'Black and female: reflections on graduate school' in *Talking Back: Thinking Feminist, Thinking Black*, London: Sheba.

Jarrett, J. (1989) 'The Experience of Black Women in British Art Schools', unpublished post-graduate diploma in Research Methodology, Middlesex University.

Johnson, C. (1985) quoted in *The Thin Black Line*, exhibition catalogue, London: ICA.

Owusu, K. (1986) *The Struggle for Black Arts in Britain. What Can We Consider Better Than Freedom?*, London: Comedia Publishing Group.

Piper, K. (1981) quoted in *The Artpack. A History of Black Artists in Britain* (1988) London: Ennisfield.

Riley, K. (1985) 'Black girls speak for themselves', in Weiner G. (ed.), *Just a Bunch of Girls*, Milton Keynes: Open University Press.

Scarman, W. G. (1982) *The Scarman Report: The Brixton Disorders 10–12 April 1981*, London: Pelican Books.

Smith (1986) *Combahee River Collective Statement: Black Feminist Organizations in the 70s and 80s*, Kitchen Table/Women of Colour Press.

Sulter, M. (ed.) (1990) *Passion: Discourses on Blackwomen's Creativity*, Urban Fox Press.

Tomlinson, S. (1984) 'Black women in higher education in Britain' in L. Barton and S. Walker (eds) *Race, Class and Education*, London and Sydney: Croom Helm.

Chapter 7

'White'[1] skins, straight masks: masquerading identities

Helen (charles)

WILL THE REAL BLACK WOMAN PLEASE STAND UP?

(Lorde 1984: 30)

These women pretended to be straight in a way that they never would have pretended to be conservative. Their political courage was far greater than their sexual openness.

(Lorde 1982: 160)

We cherish our guilty secret, buried under exquisite clothing and expensive makeup and bleaching creams (yes, still!) and hair straighteners masquerading as permanent waves . . .

Acting like an insider and feeling like an outsider, preserving our self-rejection as Black women . . .

(Lorde 1984: 170)

I lived in secrecy and rebellion. With savage social gestures I lashed out verbally at the status quo, out of hours. At work I was silent . . . and my concealed but total alienation resulted only in lack of spontaneity. I had a secret: lesbianism.

(Wilson 1988: 45)

He's invisible, a walking personification of the Negative, the most perfect achievement of your dreams, sir!

(Ellison 1965: 81)

Simulation is a Pretence of what is not, and Dissimulation a Concealement of what is.

(Sir Richard Steele (1672–1729))

CURTAIN UP

Hiding in words between spaces, the duplicitous text can be found. And concealed in the spaces between words is the subtext of desire which, for the contemporary race- and lesbian-conscious reader, offers a somewhat clandestine look into the machinations of Black American writing in the late 1920s. *Passing*, by Nella Larsen, is the catalyst for this chapter. Written in 1929, this novella captures certain essences of life-style politics which are pertinent to multi-faceted British society today. Larsen's part African-Caribbean, part Danish parentage, and her sharing of a North American cultural identity, surely informs her literary experience, creativity and thinking. Her cultural 'make-up' makes reference to the cultural 'mixed-raceness' of some Black, Asian and 'white' British people and adds to the sparse documentation of mixed-race role models. To now have access to her writings, which detail an important and rare angle from which sexuality and 'race' is positioned, is refreshing.

Readers who are alert to the subtleties of colourist and sexualist undercurrents will not be disappointed in the display of masquerade and mask with which the story is performed. The circumstances of 'race' and sexuality are intriguingly superimposed onto one another. This has triggered the enquiry of this chapter: in what way do 'race' and sexuality inform each other and how do the double codings of each premiss manifest themselves? *Passing* illustrates the juxtaposition of the always 'possible' lesbian self with the political problematizing of the Black 'I'. Sexual desire between two women protagonists is never Larsen's written certainty although it becomes a very tempting *reading* certainty. And making the protagonists' skin colour visually 'white', suggests that Larsen wishes to play the readers' understanding of entering into a discourse of Othering. A discourse which finds fodder in the slave re-memories (Morrison 1987: 35–6) of the African-American economy. A discourse, which is rooted and has emerged in Western literature since the German philosopher Hegel first deemed it a part of the Self back in the early 1800s (see Hegel 1977: 229–34; Sartre 1991). There is also a suggestion that Larsen is prompting the reader into a place where the 'I' and the 'Other' are contradictory or unfixable; where 'race' is shaken up in its own discourse and the colour of one's (political) skin can never be put down to assumption.

BACKGROUND

It is a time known as the Harlem (or Negro) Renaissance, where there was a surge in North America that placed Black arts in the spotlight. The rise is said to have begun in 1917 at the Silent Protest March in July 1917, where 10,000–15,000 Black American citizens marched to protest against the thousands of lynchings that had taken place without trial since the Emancipation Proclamation. Out of this activism came an assertion which put Black artistic recognition on a map drawn with a projection which was not (allegedly) exclusionary or distorted. Out of this projection came an era where the artistic, literary and oratorical talents of Black Americans were linked with the traditionally 'acceptable' aptitudes for song, dance, and acting. These were roles that reinforced the stereotypes of men who were feminized (Uncle Tom/Remus) or feared (the escapee); and women who were desexualized (Aunt Jemima) and over-sexualized (the lascivious mulatto).[1] It is a place in history where life-stories were written in the folds of fiction and poetry, the authors of which made possible the development of an aesthetic which could be analysed in its specificity.

But projections in the late twentieth century are looked at wryly, for it is well known that three aspects: exclusion, distortion and ignorance, have all been exercised (seemingly without exhaustion) within this 'post'-colonial era.

Taking these three aspects it is pertinent and important to explain what I mean: *Exclusion*: bearing witness to the familiar absences of women's names in the catalogue of artistic production. This absence forms a crust on the surface of resistance from those students and other scholars who are able to penetrate 'The System' and reveal (expose) the works of those who may have been tokenized, but managed to get publicized against all the odds.[2] The exclusion of women in the Harlem Renaissance is signalled by the disproportionate numbers who are actually visible. From the English (in England) student's point of view, there is only one: Zora Neale Hurston and possibly a second: Jessie Fauset.

Distortion: dominant history is an always distorting process which can only exist if accompanied by the counter-opinions of subordinate cultures. The gradual increase in, for example, alternative African, Asian, Caribbean and Cypriot histories available to schools and colleges in Britain signals the moment when they, as 'Other', push strongly against traditional British colonial history. But it is a Russian-doll syndrome. Centuries of empire-conditioning seeks not to nurture or protect, but to disengage and override. Counter-opinions and the other sides of stories jockey for a place within dominant 'white' societies and are rewarded by the gifts of 'sudden' recognition and perhaps affable welcome. And finally, *ignorance*: the inherited, transferred or borrowed silver spoon with which the blows of intentional disregard are dealt in the name of an imaginary empire.

Built on the foundations of slave expression, there existed an aesthetic in the Harlem Renaissance which produced labels that were adapted to recognize the achievements of Black people, but were also intended to undermine: educated 'negroes' were referred to as 'pseudo-primitives' by educated 'white' people (Hemenway 1986: 242), and the 'folk-people' to use Zora Neale Hurston's preferred term – or 'folk-men' to be precise – filled in the very noticeable gap in the *literati* – or 'niggerati' (Walker 1984: 88). 'New Negroes' openly and directly aimed their work at a political and wholly race-specific level but in terms of equality, there were still the old traditions of exclusion politics operating on racio-sexist levels. The anonymity of women was nurtured to the extent that even those who were not deterred from speaking (and writing) out, like Zora Neale Hurston, became part of a process of being forgotten, ignored and criticized as too 'simple' for the movement (Hemenway 1986: 241). Left to be unearthed by Black and other race-conscious writers and scholars of today,[3] it is with immense and dour curiosity that one wonders how many 'undiscovered' writers, both women and men, are strategically submerged beneath the seas of colonialist restraint.

This chapter is a British reading of a North American text. My reading is enhanced by influences of 'Blackness' derived from a mosaic of cultural backgrounds with roots in West Africa. I make no excuses for focusing on a cultural heritage (American) which I, myself, have not experienced. And I would ask readers to be aware of cross-Atlantic differences as this is useful when reading such texts as *Passing*. Mine can only be a projection of a still thwarted but highly visible form of identity which seeks to make sense of the presence of Black people in Britain – a fact which is not the same as the widespread 'settlement' of Africans in North America. There is an adage, 'we are here to stay', which infuses a sense of fightback and determination for the generations of our lives in the United Kingdom, and in some cases we are keen to follow the examples of sisters and brothers in the United States. Theirs holds the documented reinforcement of a history which begins in the same country and at the same time as the European colonization of Native American lands. As such the time-span for the economic and educational redevelopment of torn African, now African-American, cultures, is far greater than the fragmented continuity of British slave, emancipated and independent peoples in a colonialist ethos that has attempted to reproduce itself all over the world.

Becoming visible as a successful Black person in the overall artistic field is fraught with difficulties.[4] Some publishers in the United Kingdom, for example, have been known to refuse the publication of British Caribbean, Asian and African writers' work on the dubious grounds that they 'have already published Black writers from the States'. Resulting from this is the growing mythology surrounding the homogeneity of the colonized subject who happens to have been endowed 'with skin' (as opposed to being 'without skin' (Morrison 1987: 215)), which has also served to place African Blackness within the maxim of 'that without history' – as opposed to European 'whiteness' as 'that with history' – colonial history.

The cultural and historical emblems of people living under the legacy of colonization in Britain have been analysed in other writings. It is worth referring readers to the works of Homi Bhabha, David Dabydeen, Paul Gilroy, Stuart Hall, Peter Fryer, Zig Layton-Henry and Ron Ramdin, for male-centric studies, and Amina Mama, Amrit Wilson, Barbara Bush, Buchi Emecheta, Gail Lewis, Lola Young, Pratibha Parmar, Beverley Bryan and Wilmette Brown for politico-historical studies and accounts that represent women.

Returning to states of visibility offers a selection of notions related to what can be called 'the hidden'. This is denial at worst and self-preservation at best. Let me explain what I mean. At the very end of Franz Fanon's conclusion to *The Wretched of the Earth* (1963) there is a penultimate paragraph which echoes the cautionary tales of 'lily- skins'[5] and mulattos. As descendants from 'white' men who colonized African women's genitals as well as the rest of their bodies in the plantocracy, these women looked and were sometimes seen to 'behave' more 'white' than Black.

The fair-skinned were (and still are, in some cases) understood to be denying their Blackness by contravening the laws of Negro solidarity. At the same time, it could be argued that racial coalescence brought to the surface the cracks in the holistic viewing of identity implicit in these laws – cracks which would be negotiated through a strategy of pretence. But Fanon has difficulties talking about (Black) women:[6]

> Those who grant our conclusions on the psychosexuality of the white woman may ask what we have to say about the woman of color. I know nothing about her.
>
> (1986: 179–80)

The 'we' attempts a displacement of the self as writer, therefore indicating a general nescience of women of colour.

If the visibility of Black woman was problematic, what then of her visibility as lesbian? Nella Larsen offers the possibility of a dialectic here. Her fictionalizing of the position of the not-quite Black, not-quite lesbian, is manifest in *Passing*. But a return to Fanon provides a taster to the overall theme of national identity – a backgrounding of the literary analysis of *Passing*.

In *Black Skin, White Masks*, from which the title of this chapter is adapted, Fanon is talking about a specific national body – the superimposition of Black onto 'white' and vice versa. It is the diasporic shape of 'nation' for the Antillean, which has its roots in the colonial interference of the 'white' European 'scramble' for and consequent partition of Africa. Fanon's use of 'we' in his book *The Wretched of the Earth* is, nevertheless, persuasive as he sermonizes:

> . . . if we wish to reply to the expectations of the people of Europe, it is no good sending them back a reflection, of their society and their thought . . .
>
> (1963: 316)

To 'reflect' the duplicitous 'whiteness' of skin, may be observed to be an act of self-preservation or denial as illustrated above. In African-American language, the term 'passing' sketches what cannot be 'seen' by some (e.g., the referent of the person passing), but can be seen by others (e.g., those who cannot or choose not to pass). In terms of skin or racial colouring, it is more common to see film and literary references of women passing, than it is of men.[7] Comparatively, cases of 'white' people claiming

Black cultural identities in for example: dress (the 'ethnic' print, baby-carriers); hair-fashioning ('french plaits'/corn/cane-rowing, dreadlocks (see Morgan 1990)); music (reggae, rap, jazz) and so on, could be construed as a strange case in passing for Black. This only goes to show how fragmented and inconclusive dominant 'white' cultural heritages really are. What is of interest here, is the take-up of influences and the consequent self-reimaging, emanating (according to Fanon) from the newly entered dominant culture. But what of those who spend the 'best part of their lives' living in a dominant 'white' culture? In the case of members of the dominant culture borrowing images from the subordinate cultures, there is an interesting situation of reversal which incorporates a dissimulation process which makes it impossible to 'reflect' the same self-images as those belonging to the subordinate culture. This is by virtue of the fact that the continuous experience of being colonized is never acknowledged within the dominant culture and that those who make up dominant culture, itself, can only *pretend* to be subordinate.

So, the dominant culture as seasoned colonizers can be seen to backtrack into a state of pretence in order to gloss over past deeds. To colonize – whether it is a country, a culture, or clothing, is to fail to recognize that which is not offered; a plagiary which is always attempting to escape discovery.

In an essay looking at aspects of colonization in *Jane Eyre*, Gayatri Chakravorty Spivak asserts, 'the object of my investigation is the printed book, not its "author" ' (1986: 263). It would be hard to divorce writer from writing totally as what feeds the not-quite-independent analysis of a text is the always present author, disguised in the choice of wording and expression. The query, perhaps not for this chapter, is the differentiation between writer and author, or author and 'author' (see Foucault 1980). However, when the author *per se* is a nineteenth-century 'white' British woman, who is traditionally – but not without obstacles – England's canonical pride and joy, it is perhaps easier to exercise critique upon what is visible (the writing), than upon the author, who is not.

INTRODUCING THE FOREGROUND

It would be difficult to ascertain whether the writer Nella Larsen had denial or self-preservation in mind when she wrote her novella *Passing* in 1927. It would be more useful to conclude that she had both, allowing a more in-depth exploration of the vicissitudes aligned to cultural allegiance. The usual obstacles were set up before the Harlem Renaissance writer who had a vagina and not a penis. She may well have come from the 'Talented Tenth' espoused by W.E.B. Du Bois in the late 1890s, a privileged class of North Americans who, as a rule, came from free-born families and credited themselves as part of the elite and intellectual generation. Either way, Larsen, as the author of *Passing*, the text of which is the fleshing of this chapter, could easily find her way into being the object of my 'investigation'. Her nationality (Black Caribbean–'white' Danish) makes debatable comment[8] on the content of the work, in terms of its colourism or colour politics. Like Spivak, I shall concentrate on the text, leaving Nella Larsen to speak 'for herself'.

Despite the fact that Du Bois praised Larsen's writing as the 'best . . . that Negro America has produced since the heyday of Chestnutt' (quoted in McDowell 1989: 249), *Passing*, and her previous work *Quicksand*, published in 1928, got 'lost' and was not published again until 1986 in New Jersey and 1989 in London. This 'losing' of texts provides a method by which the suppressive forces of both sexism and racism merge into a practice of exclusion politics. The loss 'reflects' the image of the hidden; the non-visible 'Subordinate' that everyone knows or suspects to have existed. But the camouflage, the dissimulation, is not a prerequisite of the textual character. It merely dictates the societal positioning of those whose ancestors were slaves – whether non-memory is preferable to 're-memory' or not.

Nella Larsen's novella is divided into three parts; the first part ominously called 'Encounter' records a flashback in which Irene Redfield and Clare Kendry meet up in Chicago by chance. Irene subsequently meets Clare's colour-racist husband and a scene of humiliation and anger prompts her to sever the relationship with Clare. The second part, 'Re-encounter' takes place in New York where Irene tries to reconcile contradictory feelings for Clare. At the same time, she begins to analyse privilege in relation to skin-colour and her and her husband's position in society as middle class. A dance in Harlem makes references to the Renaissance and how powers within it lay with the 'white' classes, and Irene and Clare patch up their friendship. The third part, 'Finale', is set in winter – snow being the obvious metaphor for what lies beneath the surface of 'white' skins and straight masks. At a tea party that Irene is giving, Clare, as the uninvited guest brings betrayal, distrust and suspicion. The tables turn and, once again, Irene wishes to be rid of Clare. The contradictory feelings continue into the final scene, at a roof-top party where Clare's real identity is discovered by her husband.

Irene Redfield and Clare Kendry as joint protagonists in *Passing* furnish the reader with an encoded text. Primarily about racial skin-colour, the coding of Blackness for 'whiteness' runs parallel to a subtext of desire. To some, the subtext could be seen as lesbian. For others, something more specific in the writing would be necessary before any lesbianism emerged as an undisputed presence or occurrence.

Irene and Clare see each other for the first time since their school-days, in the Drayton Hotel's rooftop tea-room – an exclusive venue for 'white' people only. The two women, both Black and passing for 'white', keep each other's secret. Irene is greatly affected by Clare's 'seductive caressing smile' (p. 169) and general image: 'She's really almost too good-looking' (p. 156), and begins an involvement with Clare which oscillates between the indispensable literary emotions: love and hate. Their mutual interest in each other, albeit changeable, develops, and dissimulation proper begins.

An overt sexual attraction between two Black women would have borne the accusatory taboo. Lesbianism between 'white' women was still something of a non-existence in the literature of the time, although Radclyffe Hall's *The Well of Loneliness*, published at the same time (1927), can be seen as putting 'white' wealthy lesbianism on the British map. Despite the relatively more privileged circumstances of Hall, being explicit about the novel's war-scarred heroine as sexually active was still problematic. The 'undivided nights' fall between chapters of intensely descriptive writing, rendering a veiling; a hiatus in the text between the famous chapters 38 and 39. But the primary aim for Hall is to unveil lesbianism as a viable, if doomed, sexuality. What Larsen seems to be unveiling is the assertion of a 'right to desire' and a right to write about sexuality in general, as a Black or mixed-race novelist.[9] Without being dissuaded by the stereotypes of exoticism or nymphomania, or both, here was a positive move towards establishing an image of the Black self which sought to expose 'choice' as an option.

For homosexual men, such as Langston Hughes, the exposure of sexual identity proved too risky – what then of the lesbian of colour? Expressing sexualities, different from the dominant idea of heterosexuality, in the 1920s and 1930s, may have been regarded as premature for people of colour, when images of people on screen (e.g., Griffiths' *Birth of a Nation* (1915)) would have depicted mixed-race female sexuality as nymphomania (the scheming and hysterical senator's mulatto lover);[10] Black male sexuality as rape (Guy, the escapee) and 'white' female sexuality as colonizer-reproduction (i.e., the birthing of an *expanding* colonizing nation).[11] If individual investigations and exposures of homosexuality were beginning to be discussed in male 'white' literature, for example, Freud, Whitman, Wilde (all born, incidentally, in the second half of the nineteenth century, and their works were being avidly read in the first half of this century), it would not be surprising that lesbian sexuality would not have been common knowledge as part of Black women's lives. How much censorship, forced by the self or outsiders, has affected the writings of women in the Harlem Renaissance is difficult to know. One thing is clear though and that is that sexuality has been connected to Blackness as a stigmatized attribute. Imagings of Black sexuality by Black people have had to negotiate representations of the sexual self and the 'I' as the potentially assumed 'Other', and have ended up with images of reluctant compromise. Personifications of a sexual self which attempt to elude the reminiscent colonialist construction of 'Black' as degenerate, depraved and sexually over-qualified.

FOREGROUND

Clare and Irene, performing the role of being 'white' in the Drayton tea-room, are not, at first, aware that each of the 'Other' is Black. It is the first time that they see one another in twelve years, and neither of them can be sure. An interesting reversal in terms of the primary aim of passing for 'white', which is to pretend for the benefit of 'white people':

> Did that woman, could that woman, somehow know that here before her very eyes on the roof of the Drayton sat a Negro?
>
> Absurd! Impossible! White people were so stupid about such things for all that they usually asserted that they were able to

> tell; and by the most ridiculous means, fingernails, palms of hands, shapes of ears, teeth, and equally silly rot.
>
> (Larsen 1989: 150)

The irony of Irene's assumption that Clare is 'white' is never fully taken up, perhaps because one of the protagonists (Irene) would then fit (albeit temporarily) the description of 'stupid'. After more examination, an irony can be detected in Larsen's writing. The criticism of 'white' stupidity now becomes part of a criticism of Du Bois' intellectual class of Negroes, or as McDowell says, the Black middle classes (1989: 265). But this prestige can only exist in hiding and possible non-existence, for it is not the 'middle-classness' of the two women that gets them into the Drayton – it is their 'skins'.

The subtle refutation of early anthropologists' studies on Black people makes parallels with Zora Neale Hurston's own critical investigations into anthropology. These enquiries were geared to refute the conclusions made at the beginning of this century across the globe. They asserted 'structural differences' between 'white' and Black peoples (see Walker 1984: 83). The 'nature' of passing in Larsen's work hints a mockery of the anthropological 'truths' that would have been immersed in the popular mythology of the day.

The reader reads through the eyes of Irene, who sees Clare as 'An attractive-looking woman . . . with those dark, almost black, eyes and that wide mouth like a scarlet flower against the ivory of her skin' (p. 148). The over-emphasis on colour, and the colour-consciousness with which Larsen writes, is indicative of what is to follow. Larsen always describes Clare in terms of sexual attractiveness. Whether she is, at times, writing for a male or female readership is unclear, but notions of desire and the words to describe them are placed within Irene's language.

To give some examples, the word 'caress' is used frequently by Irene: 'Irene touched her arm caressingly' (p. 195); 'Irene turned away from the caress of Clare's smile' (p. 199). Here is viewed the dissimulated text in action, so to speak. As a veiling, it exercises the relative freedom for one woman to express sensual attraction for another. And the fact that it happens outside the dialogic frame, makes it a 'safe' game to play. Indeed, passing with 'white' skins and straight masks indicates a notion of the hidden which presents a failsafe mechanism – as long as the bearer of skin and mask can keep up the pretence.

If the act of writing is looked at closely, the motifs explored in this chapter can be viewed as emerging within a specific literary strategy. The moment of marking the blank page becomes, also, the moment at which a masking occurs. This may appear to contradict the themes of dissimulation and disguise in passing for 'white' and passing for straight, but it does not if the position is understood from two angles. First, dissimulation, like the blank page, does not have to be seen as a negation. It is absence relying on the fact that 'something' exists: a dual oppositional citing, which conforms to the requirements of a Western philosophy. Second, the mask indicates a hiding, which in turn transcends itself into the locality of the 'always possible' exposure, so that there is a double instanciation of clandestinity in the text: the mask in the act of hiding.

'Encounter' and 'Re-encounter' begin with a letter – the same letter – which is addressed to Irene from Clare. Melodramatic in its import, it seems to represent a staged screening of a suspense, which compliments any notion of the hidden:

> It was the last letter in Irene Redfield's little pile of morning mail . . . there was . . . something mysterious and slightly furtive about it. A thin sly thing that bore no return address to betray the sender. Not that she hadn't already known who its sender was.
>
> (Larsen 1989: 143)

The letter as unopened holds a text which is not visible. A text within a text. The unopening of the letter presents the possibility for Larsen to create a literary masking of the letter's 'author': Clare. In so doing, she fills in a deliberate gap – standing for the dissimulated blank page. The letter, too, holds a 'something'. The restaging of a flashback, a literary method from nineteenth century (women's) writing, is the gap-filler: the picture presented to the reader is of the original 'encounter' between Irene and Clare, years before.

Throughout the reading of *Passing*, it is never clear whether lesbianism, as a subtext, is a hiding, a mask, or simply is not present. It is relatively easy to give an account of *Passing* that veers towards the very definite possibility that lesbian desire is illustrated textually. Especially if the practice of selecting and isolating an extract, complete with dotted absences (. . .), is held to be an acceptable form of argument. I quote:

> For I am lonely, so lonely . . . cannot help longing to be with you again, as I have never longed for anything before . . . [my dots] and it's your fault, 'Rene dear. At least partly. For I wouldn't now, perhaps, have this terrible, this wild desire if I hadn't seen you that time in Chicago [Drayton tea-room]. . . .
>
> (1989: 145)

The concealment of words, nuances, meaning: the dissimulating begins early in the novella. By the time Clare actually appears as an 'unhidden' character, it is well into the second chapter of 'Re-encounter'. Until then, each chapter begins either with reference to two letters (both written by Clare and either unopened or on the brink of being opened), or with references to the past in flashback form.

In the Drayton tea-room flashback, Clare's 'slightly husky voice' and irresistible smiling charm (p. 150) (sur)renders Irene to the Encounter. Consecutive pages tell the story through Irene's eyes. Clare is described as 'the lovely creature' (p. 151); 'good-looking' – as mentioned previously (p. 156); Irene also has the desire to know more about her (p. 157) perhaps because she sees 'a tempting mouth' as well as 'arresting eyes, slow and mesmeric'; eyes that 'petted and caressed' Irene (p. 161). And when she hears Clare speak, she is said to have a 'voice that was so appealing, so very seductive' (p. 165).

It bears being emphasized, however, that whatever display of sexuality *is* occurring, it can only be seen to be present in the spaces between words: 'Clare had come softly into the room without knocking, and before Irene could greet her, had dropped a kiss on her dark curls' (p. 194) – this is in spite of the seeming overtness of certain textual innuendoes.

Bestowing the phrases of sensuality, depicted above, serves to posit the *notion* that 'lesbianism' was written about in the Harlem Renaissance. The most useful part of the book was discovering Deborah McDowell's 'Postscript'. Maybe the lesbian-conscious reader would find some answers there.

In her discussion, McDowell affirms the 'sexual overtones of Clare's letter'. The general analysis of the text reveals a reading which is well researched historically. As regards a reading of lesbianism inordinately linked with 'race', there was a resistance.

As a firm believer in the power of 'individual' thought, arrived at by means of 'always outside' influences, a question entered my mind. Do I doubt my own interpretation gathered on the strength of lesbian conjecture and possibility? Or do I doubt the choice and formation of McDowell's words which lie visually reinforced between the covers of Larsen's text? I did both, but the latter was more productive in terms of assessing a critical analysis as opposed to a subjective analysis.

McDowell utilizes specific quotations from Larsen's writing which, when checked with the text itself, are found to be slightly distorted. It is debatable whether this form of literary analysis is useful, and I would try to clarify the point that without *any* analysis, further development may be hindered within the 'Black feminist aesthetic' (McDowell 1986: 197); and the subject of lesbian existence may be separatized, if not tokenized, within that Black feminist aesthetic. Thus a brief enquiry into the reading of the reader/writer (McDowell) seems useful. The following quote will serve to illustrate my enquiry of McDowell's literary analysis:

> Irene tries to preserve 'a hardness from feeling' about the letter, though 'brilliant red patches flamed' in her cheeks. Unable to explain her feelings for Clare, 'for which she could find no name,' Irene dismisses them as 'just somebody walking over [her] grave.' The narrative suggests pointedly that Clare is the body walking over the grave of Irene's buried sexual feelings.
>
> (McDowell 1989: 267)

Moving through the extract, the 'blushing' of Irene's cheeks, in the light of an event which takes place later in the book, (pp. 170–4, 181) is directly symptomatic of 'humiliation, resentment and rage' (p. 145) – arguably, a sign of (lesbian) desire – but perhaps a little thwarted in the face of racist display from Clare's 'white' husband. The *nameless* 'feelings for Clare' (why dissimulate the argument of the chapter, unless there is already a doubt?) come in fact as a reference to what Irene experiences some 30 pages later, and the feelings describe a sensation of 'fear' that Irene has of Clare (p. 176). Again, this could refer to the fear of lesbian discovery but it could be argued that 'the fear' is an indication of the refusal on Clare's part to face up to her Blackness – a life-style that Irene masquerades only occasionally it seems, in rooftop tea-rooms, compared to Clare who can even masquerade as a 'white' wife.

McDowell's theory is that beneath the surface writing of racial identity 'is the more dangerous story – though not named explicitly – of Irene's awakening sexual desire for Clare' (p. 266). Because 'sexual desire for Clare' pre-empts the more descriptive term of 'lesbianism', there is the possible or probable (non)-articulated display of another notion of the hidden, which finds its place in the dominant culture's idea of safety: silencing.[12] Moving on to 'walking over my grave' (p. 176), it can be found that after an experience of acute racism dealt by Clare's 'stupid', unsuspecting 'white' husband, the passing-for-white-Irene looks incredulously into Clare's face in an attempt to understand why and how Clare could initiate and keep up the pretence in a marriage of this kind. When Clare remembers this experience in one of Larsen's dissimulated memory scenes, she uses the morbid adage to illustrate further the danger that is present as part of Clare's chosen life – and the fact that, perhaps, it could have been Irene's life.

To suggest that the grave is a veiled reference to 'Irene's buried sexual feelings' is in tune with the idea of dissimulated or closeted lesbianism, and is a tempting interpretation of the straight mask. However, it is important not to overlook the alternative (or parallel) reading which aligns itself to 'race'. The grave could be construed as an allusion to a number of things, including the passing-for-white person's desire to be 'white'.

McDowell is right to bring up the question of danger and desire, for they are repetitive in Larsen's writing. There is a problem, however, when the two themes are inadvertently linked together, and notably, when the analysis is dealing with theories of women's sexualities (see Vance 1984, esp. pp. 1–27). If Clare's incongruous death by misadventure at the end of the novella is something to go by, the motif of danger is not only literal, but also a (parodic?) statement which supports the depressing thesis that if 'lesbianism' exists as central to the twentieth-century novel, one partner needs to die (e.g. *The Threshing Floor* (Burford, 1986); *The Well of Loneliness* (Hall, 1982)) seemingly to gain sympathy from members of straight cultures. If danger is equated with desire within the domain of Black and lesbian writing, it needs to be given credence in the light of stereotypical assumptions that are made about sexual desire between same-sex partners.[13] The transgressive order of lesbianism and homosexuality makes for analyses which are not spiced with sensationalism and, thus, do not answer to the common diminutives of the voyeur. I therefore question the amalgamation of desire with danger, chiefly in the light of offensive stereotypes of Black women's sexualities being laced from the outside by images of the 'dark, unknown continent' (Africa) and as a consequence, dangerous. The licentiousness surrounding Black women *per se* is therefore desirous.[14]

On the whole, it is refreshing to read analyses which posit 'lesbianism' (or at least its possibility) as a viable sexuality for women. But a phrase like 'Clare's incredibly beautiful face' (p. 176), which falls on the same page as the 'grave' adage, might have stronger grounds for underpinning a possible lesbianism.

In her 'New Directions for Black Feminist Criticism' (1986), McDowell rightly exposes the need for a boost into a Black feminist aesthetic, particularly from Black feminist critics themselves. She acknowledges the sparsity of (Black) feminist critics and addresses her article to them. She contributes by making a criticism of Barbara Smith's article, 'Toward a Black Feminist Criticism' (1986), where she demonstrates strong criticism of Smith's interpretation of Toni Morrison's *Sula* as a lesbian novel. In accordance with the important and crucial development of feminist analysis, it is useful to have different ideas and opinions concerning (Black) textual interpretation. We must be careful though, not to patronize the type of dominancies that 'white' European cultures have entertained in the past. The 'divide and rule' ethos only leads to recolonization. As debates within a particular field increase, they necessitate a split: dividing against themselves so as to develop. But there are costs to this, as Gloria Anzaldúa maintains:

> We knew we were different . . . exiled from what is considered 'normal', white-right. And as we internalize this exile, we split apart from ourselves and each other.
>
> (1983: 169)

CURTAIN DOWN

The probability of lesbian desire between Larsen's characters remains only a probability. If Audre Lorde asks the real Black woman to stand up (see beginning of this chapter), is it an indication that the Black woman does not know who Lorde is talking to? Surely not. Pretending what is not and concealing what is, as Steele said back in the eighteenth century (ibid.), depends on ability. The 'real' Black woman, who can pass for 'white', utilizes what she has (whiteness – whatever its degree of visibility) to pretend, conceal and protect, as Larsen has shown in the depiction of her protagonists. The woman who can pass for straight, which is more common, also utilizes pretence in order to conceal.

I wanted to make use of the term dissimulation as a concept, in order to describe the various states of visibility that accompany the methodology of passing. With 'white' skins, there is much to gain in terms of access to tea-rooms. Add the mask of straight sexuality, and there is 'a guilty secret' to harbour (see Wilson 1988) in a non-accepting dominant culture.

Perhaps the secret in *Passing* is that in the 1990s, the text reveals elements of overt sexual repression within lesbian attraction. But racial repression, easily accepted as a separate and foregone conclusion (as portrayed in the title), demands critical comment:

> The Negro is universalizing him[sic]self, but at the Lycée Saint-Louis, in Paris, one was thrown out: He had had the impudence to read Engels.
>
> (Fanon 1986: 186)

The juxtapositional 'I'/'Other', with the dialectic of the straight/lesbian dynamic delineates a context within which all probabilities and possibilities can operate. But just as it is problematic to separate the writer/author from the writing/work, it is also problematic to separate the 'race' issue from the sexuality issue.

There is a difficulty in reconciling an internalized racio-homophobia. Clare Kendry's plea: '. . . I'm not safe' (p. 210) to Irene, immediately before the stupendous 'Finale', is dissimulation and clarity simultaneously. If Clare does represent a 'forbidden' sexuality and the 'unknown continent' ('race'), then notions of safety could only be used in conjunction with the transgressive Black lesbian. The interesting displacement of author for character throughout *Passing*, makes a play of where and from whom the fantasy of desire originates. Character construction via the author throws this originary desire towards the readers for final assessment, and if they are race- and lesbian-conscious they will understand, if not agree entirely, that this last quotation is both character and author simultaneously:

> Clare's ivory face was what it always was, beautiful and caressing. Or maybe today a little masked. Unrevealing. Unaltered and undisturbed by any emotion within or without.
>
> (Larsen 1989: 220)

NOTES

This essay was written in 1992.

1 The derivation of the Portuguese word 'mulatto' means a young mule, thus, a hybrid animal.

2 In the late 1980s, it was with interest that I listened to Ishmail Reed say that in the Black American literary field it is the women who rule the roost and not the men (Visiting Speaker, University of Kent 1989).

3 See, for example, Walker 1984: 84, where she tells how she 'discovered' Zora Neale Hurston's name attached to a list of mainly male literary names, like a footnote. What Walker discovers, as the research reveals more of the hostility meted out to Neale Hurston, is illustrated by this reflection:

> Would I also be attacked if I wrote and spoke my mind? And if I dared open my mouth to speak, must I always be 'correct'? And by whose standards?
>
> (1984: 87)

4 For an 'up-front' and welcome explanation of the funding and development blockages of Black women artists in Britain, see Himid 1990: 63–72.

5 I first heard this term used in Britain in the 1980s, when The Caribbean Society (University of Kent) organized for Lola Young to give a seminar on the representation of Black women in British film. The material of the seminar came from a film called *Sapphire*, made in 1959, and in the hilarious, but chilling depiction of Black women who 'looked white', extracts from the film showed them to be otherwise known as 'lily-skins'.

6 His reference to 'her' as the object case of the pronoun 'she' is in direct reference to continents and nations (e.g. Europe, Africa) only.

7 There is a reference to a 'white' man who feels more 'Black', in the television play *Chilling Out* 1989.

8 For an interesting comment on the use of prefixes ('Black', 'Negro' etc.) used in conjunction with people who do not 'belong' to dominant 'white' male Western societies, see Fanon 1986: 117.

9 For an example of Larsen's focus on women's sexual desire, see *Quicksand* published in the same volume. The following extract from

Morrison's *Beloved* illustrates well the brainwashing dealt by 'white' colonizers in terms of the viability of human sexuality:

> Slaves not supposed to have pleasurable feelings of their own; their bodies not supposed to be like that, but they have to have as many children as they can to please whoever owned them. Still, they were not supposed to have pleasure deep down. She [Grandma Baby] said for me [Denver] not to listen to all that. That I should always listen to my body and love it.
>
> (1987: 209)

10 Incidentally, the part is 'acted' in the film (*Birth of a Nation*) by a 'white' woman who fails to pass as Black.

11 The heterosexuality of 'white' men in the plantocracy very rarely reflects the substantial evidence of rape; a 'life-style' placed upon the Black (heterosexual) male as a given. This would be an interesting area for contemporary psychoanalytic investigation.

12 Adrienne Rich once wrote, 'lying is done with words, and also with silence' (1980: 186). Writers have also said that 'the writing woman is a surviving woman' and have spoken of silences as not being able to speak. Both adages speak about dissimulation. The first insists that the hidden can be represented in lying words and silence; the second implies that the writing woman does not have to be 'revealed' in terms of her gender.

13 For an example (of many) of the assumptions made about, for example, homosexual desire, see Scruton (1986) paying particular attention to chapter 9, 'Sex and Gender', and chapter 10, 'Perversion'.

14 Today the image can only answer to the stereotyping and sexist male portrayals of prostitution.

BIBLIOGRAPHY

Anzaldúa, G. (1983) 'Speaking in tongues: a letter to 3rd world women writers', in C. Moraga and G. Anzaldúa (eds) *This Bridge Called My Back*, New York: Kitchen Table: Women of Color Press.

Barthes, R. (1981) 'Theory of the text', in R. Young (ed.) *Untying the Text: A Post-Structuralist Reader*, London: Routledge & Kegan Paul.

Bryan, B., Dadzie, S. and Scafe, S. (1985) *The Heart of the Race*, London: Virago Press.

Burford, B. (1986) *The Threshing Floor*, London: Sheba.

Dyer, R. (1988) 'White', *Screen* 29 (4): 44–64.

Ellison, R. (1965) *Invisible Man*, London: Penguin.

Fanon, F. (1963) *The Wretched of the Earth*, New York: Grove Press.

Fanon, F. (1986) *Black Skin, White Masks*, London: Pluto Press.

Foucault, M. (1980) 'What is an author?' in J. V. Harari (ed.) *Textual Strategies: Perspectives in Post-Structuralist Criticism*, London: Methuen & Co.

Hall, R. (1982) *The Well of Loneliness*, London: Virago Press.

Hegel, G. W. F. (1977) *The Phenomenology of Mind*, London: George Allen & Unwin.
Hemenway, R. (1986) *Zora Neale Hurston: A Literary Biography*, London: Camden Press.
Himid, L. (1990) 'Mapping: a decade of Black women artists 1980–1990', in M. Sulter (ed.) *Passion: Discourses on Blackwomen's Creativity*, Yorkshire: Urban Fox Press.
Larsen, N. (1989) *Quicksand* and *Passing*, London: Serpent's Tail.
Lorde, A. (1982) *Zami: A New Spelling of My Name*, London: Sheba.
Lorde, A. (1984) *Sister Outsider*, New York: Crossing Press.
McDowell, D. E. (1986) 'New directions for Black feminist criticism', in E. Showalter (ed.) *The New Feminist Criticism*, London: Virago Press.
McDowell, D. E. (1989) 'Postscript' in N. Larsen (ed.) *Passing*, London: Serpent's Tail.
Morgan, Y. (1990) 'In the shade of the avocado tree, the girl next door and me', in M. Sulter (ed.) *Passion: Discourses on Blackwomen's Creativity*, Yorkshire: Urban Fox Press.
Morrison, T. (1980) *Sula*, London: Chatto & Windus.
Morrison, T. (1987) *Beloved*, London: Picador.
Rich, A. (1980) *On Lies, Secrets and Silence: Selected Prose 1966–1978*, London: Virago Press.
Scruton, R. (1986) *Sexual Desire: a 'Philosophical Investigation'*, London: Weidenfeld & Nicholson.
Sartre, J. P. (1991) *Being and Nothingness: An Essay on Phenomenological Ontology*, London: Routledge.
Smith, B. (1983) *Home Girls: A Black Feminist Anthology*, New York: Kitchen Table: Women of Color Press.
Spivak, G. C. (1986) 'Three women's texts and a critique of imperialism', in H. L. Gates (ed.) *'Race,' Writing, and Difference*, London: University of Chicago Press.
Vance, C. S. (1984) *Pleasure and Danger: Exploring Female Sexuality*, London: Routledge & Kegan Paul.
Walker, A. (1984) *In Search of Our Mother's Gardens: Womanist Prose*, London: Women's Press.
White, J. (1985) *Black Leadership in America 1895–1968*, London: Longman.
Wilson, E. (1988) 'Memoirs of an anti-heroine', in B. Cant and S. Hemmings (eds) *Radical Records: Thirty Years of Lesbian and Gay History, 1957–1987*, London: Routledge.

Chapter 8

Literature, feminism and the African woman today

Ama Ata Aidoo

> In most countries of Africa whole sectors of the economy, such as internal trade, agriculture, agro-business and health care are in the hands of women.
>
> (*West African* 9–15 September, 1991)

It might not be entirely fair to charge the development of as well-intentioned an event as Bob Geldof's Band Aid,[1] which was staged to raise both international awareness of, and funds for, Ethiopia's drought victims. But there is also no doubt that since then, the image of the African woman has been set in the minds of the world. She is breeding too many children she cannot take care of, and whom she should not expect other people to pick up the tab for. She is hungry, and so are her children. In fact, she has become an idiom of the photo-journalism of the world. In Western visual media especially the African woman is old beyond her years; she is half-naked; her drooped and withered breasts are well-exposed; there are flies buzzing around the faces of her children, and she has got a permanent begging bowl in her hand.[2]

This is a sorry pass the daughters of the continent have come to. Especially when it is considered that they are descended from some of the bravest, most independent and most innovative women this world has ever known. We speak of the Lady Tiya[3] of Nubia (*c.* 1415–1439 BC), the wife of Amunhotep III and the mother of Akhenaton and Tutankhmen, who is credited with, among other achievements, leading the women of her court to discover make-up and other beauty-enhancing processes. Tiya's daughter-in-law was of course the incomparable Nefertiti, a veritable Black beauty whose complexion was nowhere near the alạbaster she is now wilfully painted with.[4] Again from the pharonic era, we evoke Cleopatra (?69–30 BC), about whom 'more nonsense has been written . . . than about any African queen . . . mainly because of many writers' desire to paint her white. She was not a white woman. She was not a Greek . . .' says John Henrik Clarke (1981), with the impatience of painstaking scholarship in the face of half-baked ideas, prejudice and laziness.[5] According to C. W. King (London, 1872, p. 326) of Julius Caesar, Mark Antony and Cleopatra, the latter was 'the most captivating, the most learned, and the most witty . . .'. Among the many languages she spoke fluently were 'Greek, Egyptian, Latin, Ethiopian and Syrian'.[6] Yet the great William Shakespeare, heralding contemporary Western racism, could only dismiss Cleopatra as a 'strumpet' (*Antony and Cleopatra*, Act 1, Scene i).[7]

Modern Africa came into collision with Europe with the journey of Vasco da Gama (?1469–1524) travelling from Portugal southward to find Asia. He passed the Cape of Good Hope in 1496: since then Africa has never known peace. First came the slave trade, the ending of which was literally celebrated with the complete conquest and formal colonization of Africa in the middle of the nineteenth century. From then on, different Western groups considered Africa their happiest hunting ground. The energies of the people, the wealth on and inside the land – everything that could be taken was taken by some European power or other, by some groups or individual, with complete abandon. The people resisted – to the best of their abilities. But it could not have been an even match considering that, both figuratively and literally, one side was fighting with spears or bows and arrows, while the other used guns, and later, all manner of machine guns.

What is less known is that in response to Europe's insistence on conquering the continent, Africa produced, over five centuries, countless women soldiers and military strategists, many of whom died in the struggles. A famous example of these women was Nzingha (1582–1663) who tried to prevent the Portuguese from over-running her country (Angola). She died without achieving her objective. But that was after she had shown them what she was made of. On their part, the Portuguese demonstrated that they had not come to Africa on a mission of chivalry. They fought Nzingha with uncompromising ferocity and viciousness. When she suffered serious set-backs in 1645–6, they captured her younger sister Fungi, beheaded her, and threw her body into the river (Clarke 1981: 129–32).

In fact in pre-colonial times, fighting women were part of most African armies, a well-known example being the all-female battalions of Dahomey (ancient Benin; early nineteenth century), who sought to protect their empire against invaders and internal treachery. The Nzingha/Portuguese pattern was to be repeated in several areas of the continent over the following centuries. Queen after queen rose against the invaders. In the last years of the nineteenth and early twentieth centuries, Yaa Asantewaa, an Asante (Ashanti, Ghana) queen, led an insurrection against the British. Although her armies were defeated, 'it is safe to say that she helped to create part of the theoretical basis for the political emergence of modern Africa' (Clarke 1981: 132–3).

It may be granted that all these women were reigning monarchs who would therefore have found it relatively easy to organize armies against foreign occupation. But then history is also replete with accounts of insurgencies organized by women from non-monarchical traditions. An often-quoted example is the story of the women of Aba in Eastern Nigeria, who in the 1920s so successfully and collectively harassed the British that the colonial administration literally moved headquarters: from Calabar to Lagos (Emecheta, 1979). Several years earlier in Zimbabwe, Mbuya Nehanda (Nyakasikana) was accused of fomenting an insurgency against the British. In the end the conquerors decided that the only way to get rid of their fear of the woman was to hang her: and they did – in 1897.

In the years following the end of World War II, many women stayed in the forefront of the agitation for independence. In fact some, like General Muthoni (of the Mau Mau Rebellion, Kenya), became guerillas and guerilla leaders whom the enemy often feared even more than their male counterparts. Others, like Mrs Ramsome Kuti of Western Nigeria, were mainly nationalists from bourgeois backgrounds. But then, so had been the majority of the men who were their companions in such struggles.

Today we know that the story of South Africa's fight against the institutionalized horrors of conquest would be different if women – including teenagers – had not been prepared to become actively involved. And they paid the price. Many were killed, maimed, incarcerated and exiled. Sibongile Mkhabela was a student leader at the time of the Soweto riots. The only woman charged in the 7 June (1978) trials, she was jailed for three years and then banned after serving the sentence (Qunta, 1987). Countless others like Winnie Mandela, Albertina Sisulu and Zodwa Sobukwe survived the hounding of their men, only later to show an awesome readiness to carry the leadership torch with all the sacrifices such decisions inevitably entailed.

Given such a heroic tradition, it is no wonder that some of us regard the docile mendicant African woman of the last decade of the twentieth century as a media creation. On the other hand, if she did exist, then she was a mutant creation of the cumulative trauma from the last five hundred years' encounter with the West; the last one hundred years of colonial repression and denials; current neo-colonial disillusionment and denials, and a natural environment that, in many parts of the continent, was behaving almost as an implacable enemy.

> 'Someone should have taught me how to grow up to be a woman. I hear in other lands a woman is nothing. And they let her know this from the day of her birth. But here . . . they let a girl grow up as she pleases until she is married. And then she is like any woman anywhere: in order for her man to be a man, she must not think, she must not talk.'
>
> (Aidoo 1987: 112)

Critics have pointed out that although she was supposed to have lived in the latter part of the nineteenth century, the eponymous Anowa seemed to have expressed so well some of the dilemmas and concerns of the African woman today.

As I have remarked elsewhere, to a certain extent, African women are some sort of riddle. This is because, whether formally educated or not, traditional or modern, they do not fit the accepted (Western) notion of themselves as mute beasts of burden, yet they are definitely not as free and as equal as African men (especially some formally educated men) would have us believe. In fact they fall somewhere between these two notions.

What is clear, however, is that African women struggle to be independent (and articulate) at all times. I certainly hope that Nana, the grandmother of Esi in *Changes* (Aidoo 1991), epitomizes the capacity the African woman has always had to formulate clear and critical opinions in order that she would understand her position and be able to deal with it.[8] When Esi goes to consult her on whether she should go ahead and become Ali's second wife, the old lady takes her time and presents her analysis of what she sensed Esi was up to:

> 'My young lady, today you came here asking me a question. I shall try as hard as possible to give you an answer. I shall also try to make it my truth and not anybody else's . . .
>
> 'You are asking me whether you should marry this Ali of yours – who already has got his wife – and become one of his wives? Leave one man, marry another. What is the difference? Besides, you had a husband of your own, no? You had a husband of your own whom you have just left because you say he demanded too much of you and your time. But Esi tell me, doesn't a woman's time belong to a man? . . .
>
> 'Leave one man, marry another. Esi you can. You have got your job. The government gives you a house. You have got your car. You have already got your daughter. You don't even have to prove you are a woman to any man, old or new. You can pick and choose. But remember, my lady, the best husband you can ever have is he who demands all of you and all of your time. Who is a good man if not the one who eats his wife completely, and pushes her down with a good gulp of alcohol? In our time, the best citizen was the man who swallowed more than one woman. So our warriors and our kings married more women than other men in their communities. To prove that they were, by that single move, the best in the land.
>
> 'My Lady Silk, remember a man always gained in stature through any way he chose to associate with a woman. And that included adultery . . . Esi, a woman has always been diminished in her association with a man. A good woman was she who quickened the pace of her own destruction. To refuse, as a woman to be destroyed was a crime that society spotted very quickly and punished swiftly and severely.
>
> 'My Lady Silk, it was not a question of this type of marriage or that type of marriage. It was not a question of being an only wife or being one of many wives. It was not being a wife here, there, yesterday or today. The product of the womb of my womb's product, it was just being wife. It is being a woman. Esi, why do you think they took so much trouble with a girl

on her wedding day? When we were young we were told that people who were condemned to death were granted any wish on the eve of their execution. . . . Any how, a young woman on her wedding day was something like that. She was made much of, because that whole ceremony was a funeral of the self that could have been.

'Certainly from as long as even our ancestors may have been able to remember, it seemed to have always been necessary for women to be swallowed up in this way. For some reason that was the only way societies were built, societies survived and societies prospered.

'That was the only way, my grandchild. Men were the first gods in the universe and they were devouring gods. The only way they could yield their best and sometimes their worst too – was if their egos were sacrificed to: regularly. The bloodier the sacrifice, the better.

'Do I think it must always be so? Certainly not. It can be changed. It can be better . . . My Lady Silk everything is possible.'

(Aidoo 1991: 109–11)

It was important to quote her in full to enable the rationality and logic of her thoughts to unfold. It could be argued that of course with age comes wisdom. But as the Old Man in *Anowa* was quick to point out,

'It is not too much to think that the heavens might show something to children of a latter day which is hidden from them of old.'

(Aidoo 1987: 101)

Intelligence and clarity of perception does not have to come with grey hairs and wrinkles only. Sissie in *Our Sister Killjoy* was in her early twenties when she left her secure West African country to go to Europe. Yet listening to her she could see, feel and *say* a whole lot:

'Maybe I regret that I could not shut up and meekly look up to you even when I knew I disagreed with you. But you see, no one had taught me such meekness. And I wish they had.

'No my darling: it seems as if so much of the softness and meekness you and all the brothers expect of me and all the

> sisters is that which is really western. Some kind of hashed-up Victorian notions hm? Allah, me and my big mouth!!
>
> 'See, at home the woman knew her position and all that. Of course, this has been true of the woman everywhere – most of the time. But wasn't her position among our people a little more complicated than that of the dolls the colonisers brought along with them who fainted at the sight of their own bleeding fingers and carried smelling salts around, all the time, to meet just such emergencies as bleeding fingers?'
>
> (Aidoo 1988: 117)

The women in Lauretta Ngcobo's *And They Didn't Die* (1990) are no less assertive, although MaBiyela (the mother-in-law of Jezile the protagonist) and other older women in the community prove to be all too human even in their strength:

> They were capable, they were strong. They had to be. They were lonely and afraid.
>
> (Ngcobo 1990)

As a people who had to cope *daily* at the vicious end of *apartheid*, not to mention regular harassments and other provocations from the regime, they could not avoid a certain cumulative bitterness that somehow corroded their goodwill towards one another. So they were 'prone to gossip about each other's failures and misfortunes' (1990: 17).

The younger generation of women are markedly different. When pressed, they rise to the occasion with awesome courage, strength and clarity.

> The women around Nosizwe drew closer, so close that from a distance the watchful guard could not count her flagging strokes. In quick, deft movements Jezile dragged a mound of broken [stone] pieces in front of Nosizwe, a pile larger than any in front of the others. That evening, the women went back to prison happy that they had shielded her from the guard.
>
> (1990: 99)

Arrested and jailed for organizing a protest against the passes and other indignities, they cheer one another up with speeches linking their struggles to other African struggles, and prop up the weak among them.

Perhaps critics are quick to tag some of us as 'feminist' writers because we make it possible for some of our women characters to be themselves – without any of the assumed dumbness and pretended weaknesses which all societies expect from women in life and in fiction. Fair enough. However, we have to be careful with the use of the term. Simply writing about women does not make us 'feminist writers'. Making women the protagonists of novels is not feminist. Nor are men necessarily male chauvinists because they write about men. A writer is not an African nationalist simply because he or she writes about Africa and Africans. Neither is any writer a revolutionary for just writing about poor oppressed humanity. Women writers write about women because when we wake up in the morning and look in the mirror we see women. (It is the most natural thing to do.) It does not require any extra commitment – and of course, that should explain why men write about men.

Any writer's feminism comes out in her writing only when she deals with issues in ways that go beyond what would be of general interest to the author herself, as well as her potential readership. The same should be applicable to any writer and her or his ideological leanings.

Currently there is a hot and widespread debate on the issue of African women and feminism. It has become common to dismiss feminism as a foreign ideology, imported into Africa with crusading zeal to ruin good African women and stultify intellectual debate. It is also easy and a trap we all fall into every now and then to feign disinterest in the discourse. A third attitude is to maintain airily that 'we don't need feminism'. Needless to say, none of these positions are completely convincing. Even if any of them were, the implied conclusion that we do therefore not need to bother with contemporary and global forms of feminist struggles is flawed.

Feminism is an essential tool in women's struggles everywhere, and that includes African women. Every woman, as well as every man, should be a feminist. We Africans should take charge of our land and its wealth, and our own lives and the burden of our reconstruction from colonialism and slavery. If Africa is to develop, then first African women must get the best that the environment can offer for their well-being and development; in primary health care; shelter; adequate nourishment; accessibility to suitable career opportunities; freedom from sexual harassment in the workplace; freedom over their wombs, and the end to all other forms of marginalization and tokenism. For some of us, the demand from society of these fundamentals constitutes the most important element in *our* feminist thought.[9]

Nevertheless, feminism as a contemporary ideology carries other meanings and concepts of life and living – including, and especially, lesbianism. However, equating feminism with lesbianism is contentious. The latter is a sexual preference. Feminism on the other hand is an ideology, a world view, a specific notion of how life should be organized and lived by half of the entire humanity here on earth. Like all other ideologies, feminism carries its own imperatives and particular commitments.

There is a considerable lack of clarity over the significance of what it means to be lesbian. One area of specific concern is that to a number of men, and women too, the thought of women independently providing a construct to challenge the patriarchal underpinnings of *all* human society has enormous subversive implications. For such people, it is easy to equate feminism with lesbianism, and to raise lesbianism itself to a moral issue.[10]

One of the most rabid expressions of prejudice in feminist critique came out in Oladele Taiwo's *Female Novelists of Modern Africa* (1984). The book's publishers blurbed it as 'an important study', and the author himself claimed in the Preface that it is a 'celebration of the literary activities of female novelists of modern Africa'. For any writing woman, reading that 'important study' should be a sobering experience.

Taiwo manages to see the books he discusses only in one-dimensional categories. He does not attempt to do any comparative analysis. What is even more bewildering is that he treats the female authors of those novels and short stories as though they were his co-wives, to whom he dishes out his whimsical favours. He constantly remarks on their intelligence or story-telling capabilities in the best 'dancing dog' tradition.[11] For example, he declares censoriously of *Our Sister Killjoy*:

> It may be the intention of the author to prove that women can do without men in their private relationships. . . . Ms Aidoo is quite entitled to put women at the helm of affairs in her novel. But it is an error to think that they can live a full life without men.
>
> (1984: 11)

More germane to the concerns of this chapter is the fact that

Taiwo ends that particular paragraph with a solid warning: 'if such a situation is tenable in Europe, it has no chance of succeeding here [in Africa]' (ibid.). The rest of his critique comprises entirely of an attempt to scold the writers for what he suspects were all sorts of dangerous, new-fangled notions they had filled their heads with, *without his permission!* Since it is possible for an intermediary to be unfair, we should listen to Taiwo himself. To begin with, because the writers are women and as far as he is concerned all women's writing *is* 'kitchen literature', he suggests that the authors' 'economic and literary contributions and their important functions in home and family life [should be] compared with their preoccupation as novelists *to see what transfer of knowledge and skill has taken place*' (ibid., my emphasis).

Taiwo provides homilies on how to raise children, the relationship between a woman's life as a novelist and what society expects of her as a mother and the welcome outcome if such expectations are well fulfilled.

> If the correct attitude is fostered at home, in school and the community, the child has no difficulty in interacting with people and serving his nation loyally as an adult. It is only then that the mother can claim she has successfully carried out the more important obligation of parenthood, which is the proper upbringing of children.
>
> (1984: 36)

Can anything of this sort be imagined in a study of such African male novelists as Achebe, Armah, Ngugi, Mphahlele or Soyinka? Yet no woman author is spared this. Of Flora Nwapa's *Efuru*, Taiwo writes:

> In this work the novelist pursues her interest in home and family life. She portrays different kinds of marital connections in order to highlight what factors make for success or failure in married life.
>
> (1984: 26)

He comes down heavily on Buchi Emecheta, author of *The Joys of Motherhood*:

> The novelist's treatment of polygamy is uninspiring. By making Nnaife so completely ineffective as the head of the extended

> family she may be suggesting that polygamy is one of the traditional practices which need to be changed.
>
> (1984: 184)

And yet this traditionalist view is nothing compared with the baffling insensitivity exposed in his comments on the work of Southern African novelist Bessie Head (e.g. 1969; 1971; 1973):

> Why does a man like Makhaya not stay on and fight the system from within, instead of fleeing to another country? . . . one does not change . . . 'false beliefs' by running away from the situation which they have helped to generate.
>
> (1984: 44–5)

How can any African in the early 1980s manage to arrive at the conclusion that the Black people in South Africa helped to 'generate' *apartheid*? Would such a dismissive approach to the context of the works be permitted if the authors were male? It seems that Taiwo's main concern is to put women in their place. Indeed, he as good as asks them how they came to dare to write at all, complaining that each of the women writers produces work that is 'packed full of women'! In other words, men should write about men, and women, if they want their works to be considered 'literature', should also have male protagonists.

Maybe one should hasten to add at this stage, that as writers we are not looking for approbation. What we have a right to expect is that commentators try harder to give our work some of their best in time and attention, as well as the full weight of their intelligence and scholarship. In this regard Vincent Odamtten has made a very impressive and ground-breaking contribution with his study of my work *The Developing Art of Ama Ata Aidoo: Reading Against Neo-colonialism* (1992). Not only does he give the texts a close reading, but he also treats their contents seriously, with the result that he arrives at profound insights into the material itself, contemporary African literature and, indeed, literature generally.

WRITING ABOUT WOMEN

'Why do you write about women?'[12] This is the question which all interviewers for the print and electronic media, and all manner of researchers invariably ask any woman writer. The only honest answer to which should of course be the counter question: 'Whom else should we women writers write about?'

Since deep down in every-one's soul (including the souls of women freelance journalists and researchers), there is the conviction that even women writers must write about men, the logical conclusion therefore is that when a woman writes about women, it is abnormal – it is because she is a feminist. From all of which we conclude that *any writing that focuses attention on women is feminist literature.* Of course this is unfair, wrong and false. But it is also the central reality in popular notions about 'feminist writing'.

Perhaps it was with such considerations in mind that Alice Walker (1984) opened the latest and most interesting front in the discourse when she proposed that we substitute for 'feminist' the term 'womanist' to describe global African women's particular concerns. Titled *In Search of Our Mother's Gardens*, Walker subtitled her seminal essays on 'Black' women – especially African-Americans – *Womanist Prose.* The terminology has since then been seriously taken up on three continents.

In her contribution to the debate, Chikwenye Okonjo Ogunyemi writes:

> More often than not, where a white woman may be a feminist, a black woman writer is likely to be a 'womanist'. That is she would recognise that along with her consciousness of sexual issues, she must incorporate racial, cultural, national and political considerations into her philosophy.
>
> (1985)

In *Diverse Voices*, Caroline Rooney (1991) is critical of Ogunyemi for assuming a 'polarisation of the two positions in terms of "white" and "black" ', although Rooney grants that Ogunyemi's 'distinction between feminism and womanism is a useful and broadly apt one'.

Yet the problem really is not the polarization Rooney and other 'white' feminists seem to be so worried about. African women did not create the polarization. It is a historical fact based on the realities of Africa's conquest by Europe and the consequent enslavement of her peoples in the Americas, the Caribbean and on the continent of Africa: the latter normally and euphemistically described as 'colonization'. This fact created a major schism in the fortunes of African and European women which must inevitably haunt the relationship of the two groups for a very long time to come.

The situation is not improved by the arrogance with which some 'white' feminists handle current feminist discussions. In October 1988 a persistent nightmare became reality in an incredible scenario in Hamburg, where a group of African writers had been invited to a workshop organized by Werkstatt, entitled 'Days of African Literature'. One of the panels had been dedicated to issues about African women and African women writers. It soon became apparent – after the panelists had made their statements and the discussion had been opened to the floor – that on the question of the status of African women in their own societies, the audience was split into two clear factions.

On one side were European feminists who were almost bullying us, the African women and African women writers on the panel, to declare for their brand of feminism. The European feminists, it seemed, knew much more about the oppression of African women than the African women writers who had been flown all the way from wherever they had been, ostensibly to inform the conference about themselves and their environment. In fact, one woman had come out to say openly that 'you bourgeois African women are in no position to speak for the ordinary African woman in the village.' Naturally, it had not struck her that it was even more ridiculous that she, a bourgeois European woman, was trying to speak for 'the ordinary African woman in the village'. Colonial legacies and all!

Another part of the audience was made up of African male students, workers and professionals who, it turned out, had also come to the meeting with a clear-cut mission; to order the African women writers to say that we did *not* want feminism at all in Africa. Because after all, African men also knew better when it came to what the African woman in Africa needed: whatever that was, it definitely did not include feminism!

In the end, out of sheer exasperation, we had to tell both the European feminists and the African men resident in Europe that, strange as it might seem, African women (including we African women writers) are quite capable of making up our own minds and speaking for ourselves.

The tragedy of the non-communication between some African women and the European feminists seemed to have finally bloomed around Mineke Schipper's book: *Source of All Evil* –

African Proverbs and Sayings on Women (1991). The cover of the book, its sub-title, the dedication, not to mention the editing of the proverbs: it seemed there was not a single aspect of the book that did not hurt some African sensibility or other.

In response to a message I sent to Schipper objecting to her decision to dedicate the book to me and to two other African writers, she sent me a letter in which she said, among other lines of defence, that 'a dedication is a gift to somebody you feel close to. Other books I dedicated to my parents, my husband, my children, dear old friends . . .'. She also went on to say how much she admired 'my strength' and other aspects of my personality, and to mention other Africans she had previously dedicated books to. In the end, I felt the issues being raised were so important, I should put my views down. The decision crystallized in what finally became an open letter to her, of which the following comprised the main text:

'*Dear Mineke*

Re: Source of All Evil – African Proverbs and Sayings on Women

. . . My feeling of unease about your book or rather the title and sub-title is very concrete. That is why I also felt unhappy about the dedication to me, Micere [Mugo] and Miriam [Thali]. This does not in any way mean that I am unaware of the importance of authors deciding to dedicate their books to people they love or respect. After all, and especially for many of us writers who often do not have much else of value, dedicating our books is the highest demonstration of appreciation we can offer. And as you may be aware from my books, I do it all the time. Nor do I, in this particular instance, doubt the genuineness of the sentiments behind your gesture.

However, for a number of years now, some of us have been getting more and more convinced that somehow, the European (or Western) woman believes that her position in society is the highest of all women's positions in the world. That conversely, the position of the African woman in society is the lowest. This is in line with the normal European way of looking at Africa and Africans. It is also a dichotomy of conquest. You are the conquerors. We are the vanquished. It stands to reason then that you should represent the superior and we the inferior in all things. The only problem arises when, as now, this belief threatens to become a cornerstone of Euro-Western feminism, and one is either being pressurised to endorse it or just used to endorse it.

For years, some of us have been struggling to get the world to look at the African woman properly. Hoping that with some honesty it would be seen that vis-á-vis *the rest of the world, the position of the African woman has not only* not been *that bad, she had been far better off than others. That when the African woman's position fell into the pits it was as a result of colonial intervention. Mineke, I may be wrong, but I suspect that any* traditional *African woman would be aghast contemplating the evidence of other people's dehumanisation of women: from the complete depersonalisation of the woman through name-change after marriage which was invented only in nineteenth century Europe (can you imagine)?! and now slavishly copied around the world, to foot-binding in China and widow-burning in India. At the very least, I hope we could agree that the African woman never went through worse.*

So what hurts about your book or its title and sub-title is that they reaffirm the prejudices we are struggling so hard to change. And from someone like you, that is really quite unforgivable. Surely, a scholar of your standing cannot be unaware that almost any data from any research can be manipulated to tell any tale we would want told, depending on our aims and objectives? Or that perhaps, even more than any other material, proverbs are highly susceptible to such manipulation? Had you considered the very different impression you would have created if you had titled and sub-titled your book differently, using some other proverb from even your highly selective compilation? 'Mother is Gold[13] – African Proverbs and Sayings about Women' *for instance? But of course, your aim was not to supply your readers with* positive *ideas about women from Africa.*

Plainly put Mineke, I am just tired of the way Africa always surfaces first whenever there is something negative on someone's agenda.

I am happy for you that UNESCO has adopted the project. But you see, the African opening was necessary. Or wasn't it? With those kinds of title and sub-title, I genuinely think that it would have been more valid if you had begun the project

> *from your own society. You could have laid the foundation with Dutch and European negative sayings about women, and then moved out to the rest of the world in search of parallels among other peoples: including Africans*'
>
> (30 January 1992)
>
> [The letter ends with the normal good wishes and new year greeting.]

I go on to discuss what could or could not be done with the offending dedication, and thank her for the copy of the book which, I note, 'makes very interesting, if quite often controversial reading'.

Ironically, a few days after sending off the original of my letter to Schipper, I came upon a review of *Source of All Evil* by Ifi Amadiume (1991–92) in which, uncannily, she expressed sentiments similar to those in my letter, *and more.*

The review begins by drawing attention to the fact that in the book's blurb, Schipper is described as an 'internationally known expert on Third World Literature'. Amadiume then proceeds to challenge a few of Schipper's philosophical positions including the latter's concept of truth, quoting an Igbo proverb to support her point. She goes on to assert that:

> there cannot be a male monopoly on the use of proverbs as the authors suggests . . . I therefore read the book with unease, feeling that the author . . . objectified women as a thing to be commented on.
>
> (1991–92)

Amadiume also queries Schipper's methodology and epistemology. She points out the 'indomitable power of African women . . . their ability to answer back, countering silence', and then adds with thinly veiled contempt: 'a subordinate tongue-tied European white woman can hardly understand this characteristic'. This final sentence of the paragraph sums up what some African commentators believe to be a major difference between some African women and some of their European counterparts.

Amadiume is clear:

> Schipper obviously has not taken heed of the Black/African women's arguments against white women's ethnocentrism and imperialism, or else, the Eurocentric conclusions on the universal subordinate status postulated by Rosaldo and Lamphere

(in *Women, Culture and Society*, 1974) would not have been reproduced uncritically in 1991.

(1991–92)

What seems to emerge from both my letter and Amadiume's review is unmistakable: some sectors of contemporary African society are beginning to express the long-suppressed feelings of irritation and exasperation with the cavalier use of African artistic objects, and other creative data, by sundry European (Western) happy hunters in Africa. And maybe, we came out not a day too soon!

NOTES

1 Also sometimes referred to as 'Live Aid', Geldof organized the concert in 1985: it galvanized the world. Among the honours Geldof received was a knighthood bestowed by the queen of England, and the 1986/87 Third World Prize. The Western media consequently fell over itself to pay him a well-deserved homage, calling him 'Santa Bob', 'Sir Bob', and 'Saint Bob'.

2 This picture is the first part of a tri-focal image the media gives the world of Africa. Travel agents, holiday tour operators and airlines insist on two others: both of them to do with nature. So the second Africa we see is the land of exotic flora, and vanishing fauna, for example the threatened elephant and the black rhino. Then finally we get the Africa of 'golden' beaches, great lakes against crimson sunsets, calm rivers, breathtaking waterfalls, and *always*, white folks having fun! The press in Africa is no better.

3 Sometimes spelt Tiy*e*, she was often hailed as '. . . the Princess, the most praised, the lady of grace, sweet in her love, who fills the palace with her beauty, the Regent of the North and South, the Great Wife of the King who loves her, the lady of both lands, Tiye . . .'.

4 Or the two-tone image of her on the 20 pfenning stamp which the city of Berlin insists on insulting her with!

5 *Black Women in Antiquity* is the source for all quotations on the women of ancient times mentioned in this chapter. See also other volumes in *The Journal of African Civilizations* series edited by the same – a true labour of love which van Sertima has kept going for years at Rutgers University, with no reward or recognition. In fact there is something quite interesting here. The earlier work on classical Egypt by van Sertima, Cheikh Anta Diop (e.g. *Cultural Unity of Negro Africa* (1980)) and other people of African descent were also completely ignored. 'The world' seemed to have begun to believe that Egypt *was* African and Black, only since Martin Bernal's *Black Athena: The Afroasiatic Roots of Classical Civilization* (1987).

6 Cleopatra was supposed to have been an 'illegitimate offspring of Ptolemy XI' which supposition presumably lends her the whiteness.

Again if it was true, how could a royal princess of the pharaohs be the illegitimate offspring of a Greek king? Did dynastic marriages not exist then? Or are we just transposing our latter-day racism on to an age that possibly did not suffer from this particular mental, psychological and spiritual sickness? A fuller comment on this issue is urgently called for.

7 Shakespeare was unbelievably crude about Cleopatra. But then, the Bard's racism is becoming a great source of the most acute embarrassment. See also *The Tempest, The Merchant of Venice, Titus Andronicus*, and most especially *Othello*.

8 I firmly believe that it is not only academics who can rationalize or do analysis. Formal education and training only sharpen our basic intellect and allow us a certain breadth of field for comparison.

9 Much of this paragraph quotes or paraphrases 'Changing relations between the sexes in the African experience – a quick look at the status quo': a paper I presented in a keynote address to a conference organized by the Forum of African Students (FAST) at York University, Toronto, in October 1989.

10 This view would be countered however by many Black and 'white' lesbian and gay writers. For a discussion of lesbianism as an ideological stance, and the connections between feminism and lesbianism see Lorde (1984); Abelove *et al.* (1993); Rich (1980). (DJM, ed.)

11 This is a reference to a general attitude that views women performing in any capacity normally only expected of men, as being almost as strange as 'a dog's walking on his hind legs. It is not done well, but you are surprised to find it done at all'! (Dr Johnson, quoted by Virginia Woolf in *A Room of One's Own*).

12 I have been asked this almost every time – everywhere and by everyone I have been interviewed by. In fact, in response to the incessant questioning, I felt compelled to do a paper titled 'Why women writers write about women' which I first presented at the University of Richmond in 1989. But then I had to relive the nightmare over and over and over again, when I was in London for the production of *Anowa* at the Gate Theatre, and to promote *Changes* which had just come out in April/May 1991.

13 The whole proverb is 'mother is gold, father is mirror' (Yoruba, Nigeria).

BIBLIOGRAPHY

Abelove, H. *et al.* (eds) (1993) *The Lesbian and Gay Studies Reader*, London and New York: Routledge.

Aidoo, A. A. (1987) *The Dilemma of a Ghost and Anowa*, Harlow: Longman.

Aidoo, A. A. (1988) *Our Sister Killjoy or Reflections from a Black-eyed Squint*, Harlow: Longman.

Aidoo, A. A. (1991) *Changes – A Love Story*, London: The Women's Press.

Amadiume, I. (1991) 'Ammunition for the misogynist', *African World Review*, Oct. 1991–Mar. 1992.
Bernal, M. (1987) *Black Athena: the Afroasiatic Roots of Classical Civilization*, New Brunswick NY: Rutgers University Press.
Clarke, J. H. (1981) 'Black women in antiquity' in I. van Sertima (ed.) *Black Women in Antiquity*, New Brunswick NY: Rutgers University Press.
Diop, C. A. (1980) *Cultural Unity of Negro Africa*, London: Karnak House.
Emecheta, B. (1979) *Joys of Motherhood*, London: Allison & Busby.
Head, B. (1969) *When Rain Clouds Gather*, London: Heinemann.
Head, B. (1971) *Maru*, London: Heinemann.
Head, B. (1973) *A Question of Power*, London: Heinemann.
Lorde, A. (1984) *Sister Outsider*, New York: Crossing Press.
Nwapa, F. (1966) *Efuru, Heinemann.*
Ngcobo, L. (1990) *And They Didn't Die*, London: Virago.
Odamtten, V. O. (1992) 'The Developing Art of Ama Ata Aidoo', doctoral thesis presented to the State University of New York, New York.
Ogunyemi, C. O. (1985) 'Womanism: the dynamics of the Black female novel in English', *Signs* II(1), Autumn.
Qunta, C. (1987) *Women in Southern Africa*, Heinemann.
Rich, A. (1980) *On Lies, Secrets and Silence*, London: Virago.
Rooney, C. (1991) 'Are we in the company of feminists?' in Jump, H. D. (ed.) *Diverse Voices*, London: Harvester Wheatsheaf.
Rosaldo, M. and Lamphere, L. (eds) (1974) *Women, Culture and Society*, Stanford: Stanford University Press.
Schipper, M. (1991) *Source of All Evil: African Proverbs and Sayings on Women*, London: Allison & Busby.
Taiwo, O. (1984) *Female Novelists of Modern Africa*, London and Basingstoke: Macmillan.
Walker, A. (1984) *In Search of Our Mother's Gardens: Womanist Prose*, Harcourt Brace Jovanovich.

Chapter 9

The rough side of the mountain: Black women and representation in film

Lola Young

Women of African descent have played central roles in the development of Western Euro-capitalism as (among many other roles) producers, 'breeders', labourers and wet-nurses. When it comes to film roles in Euro-American media, however, they are scarcely in evidence. Why is this the case?

Colonial, neo-colonial and imperial discourses have conceptualized Western European culture, experience and consciousness as being located at the centre of the world. In Joseph Conrad's much critiqued novella *Heart of Darkness*, we learn a little of the kind of sensibility that left unquestioned the role of 'white' people in shedding 'light' (read truth, knowledge, civilization) into the 'dark' (read atavistic, savage, mysterious) corners of the world. *Heart of Darkness* begins by explaining the central protagonist's predilection for travelling:

> 'Now when I was a little chap, I had a passion for maps. I would look for hours at South America, or Africa, or Australia, and lose myself in the glories of exploration. At that time there were many blank spaces on the earth, and when I saw one that looked particularly inviting on a map (but they all look like that) I would put my finger on it and say, "When I grow up I will go there".'
>
> (Marlow, in Conrad 1989)

Even as a small child, Marlow has a naturalized sense of his superiority as a European, an awareness that he has the right to roam the world filling in the 'blank spaces' with his presence. The blank spaces, the fantasized 'darkness' of the continent of Africa appear as places where he can gratify his desire to both lose his identity and to affirm it. Reading Africa as a 'blank space', a 'dark continent' waiting for Europeans to illuminate its furthest reaches, allowed 'white' people to conceptualize and interpret the land and its people according to their projective fantasies.

As the embodiment of those fantasies, Black people have been expected to behave, respond and experience in particular ways: we are 'obliged' to play particular roles. In the case of most 'white' authored fictional narratives this means being confined to specific spheres of action.

My earliest remembered experience of the limitations placed on Black people by 'white' people's racism was when I first went to school at the age of five. Far from being in a position of 'putting my finger' on a blank space and claiming it as my own, I was the dark blankness come to a North London primary school in the mid-1950s. I was a novelty and the children in my class would boast to their less fortunate peers that they had a 'coloured girl', a 'darkie from Africa' in the class. More distressing than this early experience of the power of fantasy and exoticism was the consistency with which I was chosen to play the witch every play-time. That childhood re-memory was reinvoked, when as a professional actor during the mid-1980s I was cast as one of the three witches in a production of *Macbeth* at the Young Vic in London. That experience was not without its contradictions since for many years, Black actors have demanded the right to play as wide a range of characters as 'white' actors are allowed to, and here was I stuck playing a witch again, albeit in Shakespeare.

The casting of Black people in anything other than contemporary urban-based drama causes a paroxysm of anxiety amongst drama critics, and the appropriation of Shakespearean roles makes for even more uneasiness than usual. There were some particularly virulent attacks on the concept of integrated casting in the broadsheets at the time, I remember. My characterization of a witch did not raise any specific comment: perhaps a raggedly dressed Black female heralding death and disorder was acceptable in *that* play. Black hags and whores are permissible, but Black people's appropriation of Shakespeare – the ultimate icon of English logocentric culture and heritage – is considered to be an outrage.

The furore that such casting provoked seemed to me to be excessive: I could only regard it as a symptom of an irrational psychopathology. All that those of us in the company who cared were able to vocalize were cries of 'these critics are racist' – knowing that this was by no means an adequate response, but feeling unable to understand and articulate beyond that.

Eventually, the prospect of playing the Black Woman's repertoire – bus conductor, nurse, prostitute – in an endless loop for the rest of my life led me to abandon the world of Equity meetings, humiliating auditions, sitcoms and hospital dramas. However, there are two significant questions raised by these acting experiences which feed into my current work. First, why are Black women and men confined to particular roles and how might a critique of that stereotyping be articulated? Second, what is it within 'white' people's cultures that manifests itself in the Fanonian terms of 'negrophobia' and 'negrophilia'? (Fanon 1986).

This chapter is motored by these questions and is an attempt to raise yet more, by asking why 'white' feminist academic film criticism – which has explored gender and heterosexuality at length – has been deployed in such a way as to efface its ethnocentrism. As Black people increasingly engage with academia, the issue of the appropriateness of Eurocentric academic discourse to the study of Black texts and cultural criticism has become a site of intense speculation and contestation. Ethnocentrism is a defining characteristic of a vast body of European and Anglo-American theoretical writing and it is important for Black cultural commentators and analysts to respond by critically engaging with that material. I want to suggest ways of using psychoanalytic theory in particular, to help unravel some of the complexities of 'race', gender and representation.

As I have indicated, the act of critical reassessment is a consistent and necessary feature of Black cultural criticism: established theoretical frameworks need to be destabilized and recast in terms of 'race', and the historical determinants of relationships between Black and 'white' people. In his essay, *The New Cultural Politics of Difference*, Cornel West (1992) identifies a number of crucial projects to be undertaken by Black cultural workers which indicate the necessity of deconstruction for the purposes of reconstruction:

> Black cultural workers must constitute and sustain discursive and institutional networks that . . . demystify power relations that incorporate class, patriarchal and homophobic biases, and construct more multi-valent and multi-dimensional responses

that articulate the complexity and diversity of Black cultural practices in the modern and postmodern world.

(1992: 29)

West also discusses stereotypes, and the notion of negative and positive imagery, and argues that the question of representations and their relationship to the referent is a tricky one in which nothing can be taken for granted.

The idea that the European has the right to define and determine the status of the Other is pervasive and the resulting misrecognitions are legion. Robert Goldwater cites an important cultural moment in recounting how, when 'white' explorers showed the people of the Kalahari photographs that had been taken of them, the San[1] did not recognize these apparently life-like, apparently accurate representations of their selves (Goldwater 1987).

When looking at most images of Black women on film, many of us are also troubled and find it difficult to equate what we see with what we 'know'. This perplexity may be located in the 'knowledge' that the reality of Black women's lives is somewhat different to the way in which it is represented – but what is meant by that? The position which considers Black women to be 'misrepresented' in mainstream cinema is problematic because such a stance implies that the answer to the constant parade of negative stereotypical images of Black women is to produce a 'truthful' or realistic representation of Black women. In demanding an end to 'negative' images of Black women, the notion of a 'Real Black Woman' is being invoked. The implication here is that as Black women we may claim unmediated access to an essential Black female subject: of course, that woman exists in the realms of mythology only. Nevertheless, on a day-to-day basis, for tactical reasons, it is absolutely necessary to argue against demeaning portrayals of Black women and men, whether they appear in 'white'- or Black-authored texts. The contestation of offensive stereotypes and the refusal to accept emblematic and stereotypical characterizations is of strategic value and part of a strategy for psychological and cultural survival.

There is a problem though in analysing the issues in this way in the long term since the invocation of 'the authentic Black woman' may take an essentialist turn and end by accepting, and colluding with, the same oppressive system which we seek to undermine and dismantle: a system based on an essentialism which denies the historical, material and political predicates of culture and the experiences and effects of oppressing and oppression.

In any case, the issue is not simply a question of real Black women being misrepresented but of cinematic discursive practices sustaining particular perspectives on what a Black woman is. If we accept, as feminists have argued, that cinematic forms connive in reproducing the ideology which underpins patriarchy, then we must also recognize cinema's complicity in the naturalizing of power relations between Black and 'white' people.

There is another aspect of the representation problematic – the dependence of 'white' identity on the notion of its normality and its supremacy. Again, Cornel West is clear about the analytical task that Black critics face and urges that we:

> must investigate and interrogate the other of Blackness – Whiteness. One cannot deconstruct the binary oppositional logic of images of Blackness without extending it to the contrary condition of Blackness/Whiteness itself.
>
> (1992: 29)

The study and analysis of racial and cultural identity has come to revolve around 'Blackness' as the object of fascination (desire?) leaving unspoken issues of 'white' ethnicity, 'Whiteness' as the unarticulated norm. As Coco Fusco (1988) has pointed out, 'to ignore white ethnicity is to redouble its hegemony by naturalizing it. Without specifically addressing white ethnicity, there can be no critical evaluation of the construction of the other.'

In regard to academic film criticism, where feminist analyses of gender and representation have been highly influential, 'whiteness' is at once effaced and universalized. Issues of ethnicity and 'race' have rarely been consistently addressed by 'white' feminist academics: this has been a significant and shameful gap in theoretical considerations of gender and sexuality in film criticism for far too long. There are a number of reasons why this situation exists, some of which will be touched on in this chapter, although it is an issue which deserves much more detailed exploration than I can give here. The histories of racism, of colonialism and slavery, of notions of femininity and feminism itself, are intimately connected: 'race' and racism are implicated in conceptualizations of 'woman' and the 'feminine' and thus feminism, but these issues are most frequently latent and left unspoken by 'white' feminists. These repressed histories and their links are available for analysis in a range of historical and contemporary cultural images (see e.g. Ware 1992). So far, however, it has been largely left to Black womanists/feminists to struggle constantly for a constructive critique of the power relations embedded in 'race', class and gender issues (see Hill Collins 1991).

What, then, are the historical and cultural determinants of the on-screen relationships between Black and 'white' women, and how do representations of Black female sexuality connect with colonial history and the socio-sexual hierarchies established during slavery and colonialism? The answers to these questions may help us to understand why it is that the number of Black female characters on film is still insignificant, and why most 'white'-authored films are underpinned by narcissism, a naturalized sense of racial superiority, and a particular set of disavowed sexual anxieties provoked by the fantasized sexuality of the African Other. I want now to map out some important historical relationships between Black and 'white' men and women which have fed into current notions of racial and sexual difference and the representation of these facets of human subjectivity.

DARK CONTINENT/'WHITE' MAN'S BURDEN

Given the ways in which African sexual Otherness was inscribed into colonialist medical/scientific, literary and photographic discourses, the perpetuation of the fantasy of Black sexuality through the medium of film was inevitable. Film obviously privileges the visible, and it is the visibility of racial difference – of Blackness – that makes it such a potent signifier of racial and cultural Otherness. Sander Gilman (1985) notes that in constructing a representational system for the Other, visible, physical signs of difference are sought out: skin colour and physiognomy are identified as being the antithesis of the idealized 'white' self. These judgements about difference may apply to skin colour and facial features but also to anatomical sexual structures such as the shape of the genitalia. 'Deviations' from the so-called norm become labelled as pathological and directly linked with perverse sexuality and 'race'. The linkage is elided, and the mere sight of the Other may be enough to evoke the disgust, fear and anxiety associated with deviance, disease and sex: Fanon (1986) named this collection of anxieties about Black people 'Negrophobia'.

European fantasies about the sexuality of Black people were consolidated during the period of colonial expansion. When European men encountered tribal kinship structures based on polyandry they viewed these familial practices as an expression of excessive Black female sexuality which was to be both conquered and economically exploited. These are the terms on which European men founded their relationship with Africa and its women. Although the 'white *man's* burden' was actually *his* sexuality and its control, under slavery and colonialism Black female sexuality was to be both tamed and capitalized (Gilman 1985).

In imperial literature, Africa itself is referred to as female – with all the contradictory connotations of passivity, uncontrollability, desire and danger. Freud's description of European women as the 'dark continent' (1986a: 313) suggests the potential danger of 'penetrating' and being 'swallowed up in the interior', as well as the mystery and the unknowableness of Woman – and embodies it in the colonial metaphor.

The African woman functioned as a contrast by which the European male could conceive of his self as fearless, active, independent, in control, virile and so on. Black women were seen as not-male, but neither were they women in the same sense as 'white' women were: they were dehumanized and deprived of gender. Under the oppressive institution of slavery African females were at once women (sexualized, reproductive, subordinated) and not-women (not 'feminine'; not pure; not fragile; sexually available).

The European woman was idealized and symbolic of the plantocrats' control – of Self, of Others – and her femininity was made distinctive from that of the African woman and the European woman of the 'lower' social orders. Both of these groups of women – Black and lower-class 'white' (especially prostitutes) – were pathologized but they were also a source of illicit sexual pleasure for many European men. The African woman's body was a site of ambivalence for the male Euro-supremacist, evoking as it did fascination, fear, desire, anxiety and guilt; the anxieties instigated by sexual difference exacerbated by 'race'.

The 'white', middle-class male – in the powerful position of 'definer' of norms – projected his own anxieties in the realm of sexuality on to icons of Otherness; Black people, working-class people or women. 'White' men fantasized that Black men had large penises, and having projected the anxiety about their potency on to the African, the male Euro-supremacist then had to act on it as though it were an external reality. Thus Black manhood was imagined as a threat to 'white' womanhood, since possession of the large penis potentially allowed the African to give sexual satisfaction to the European woman that he (the 'white' male) could not. Fearing that he was unable to give 'his' woman what she wanted (her sexual appetite conceptualized as threatening to devour him, her sexuality dangerous, mysterious and inaccessible) he idealized 'white' feminine purity and delicacy and placed her on a pedestal: at the same time he punished the African, for supposedly daring to usurp his place through the literal and figurative castration of the Black male. In the case of both females and males, the contention that Blacks were oversexed is historically linked to, and 'proven' by, alleged anatomical excesses of the genitalia and reproductive organs.[2]

For the 'white' woman in this complex set of relations, her dissatisfaction with the way in which she was sexually situated frequently prompted jealousy of the slave woman who was forced to be sexually available to 'white' males. This failure of 'white' women to connect their oppression under patriarchy to the Black woman's oppression through racism was encouraged by the plantocratic male through the ideology of racial superiority.

The traces of this colonial history are evident in film texts where Black people are annihilated, criminalized and labelled as sexually aberrant: where their sexual behaviour is monitored and regulated to a high degree. Representations of Black people on screen function as comforters, helping to maintain 'white', middle-class identity as synonymous with power, control and autonomy. The illusory identity needs constant reassurance of its imagined supremacy and centrality, and cultural narratives which perform this function. This security is, of course, spurious and constantly under threat because it is in reality highly dependent on its fantasized conceptualizations of Otherness to sustain that sense of security, of preeminence. In film, fictions are continually created which preserve the narcissistic illusion of the centrality of 'white', masculine, middle-class identity. This results in the predominance of 'white' male protagonists in most film narratives. Representations of 'white' women often serve to shore up and legitimate this narcissism.

BLACK WOMEN'S BUSINESS? PSYCHOANALYSIS, FEMINISM AND 'RACE'

Feminist cultural theory and criticism has been castigated for its lack of attention to ethnicity: in regard to film theory, the problem has been located in feminism's contentious and contested relationship with psychoanalysis. Before I embark on a psychoanalytically informed analysis of Whoopi Goldberg's role in *Ghost* (Jerry Zucker (dir.) 1990), I would like to indicate a number of approaches to some of the problems which have been identified in applying such a method of 'race' and textual analysis.

It has been suggested by Jane Gaines (1988), that a materialist approach to racially differentiated representation would be more productive than feminist theorists' emphasis on psychoanalytic interpretations of texts because the stress on sexual difference has led to a privileging of gender as the locus of oppression. As Gaines forcefully argues, materialist explanations of racism are a crucial component of any holistic analysis involving 'race'. However, such arguments are insufficient on their own: there are distinct limitations to the consideration of racism as the product of the economic structure of Western societies. It is, of course, politically essential to analyse racism as a strategy of capitalism, and to analyse the way in which it is institutionalized and systemic, but this alone is not able adequately to clarify how power relations embedded in textual systems and forms of representation may be unconsciously sustained.

The question of what racism is, and its inter-relationship with other forms of oppression, needs to be unpacked since single-focus analyses have – for the most part – provided inadequate explanatory models for examining the position of Black women in culture.

It is fruitless to argue over whether the most divisive aspect of subjectivity is 'race' or gender. As socialized human beings we learn what masculinity and femininity, dominance and oppression mean in the context of the class and ethnic background in which we grow up. We do not learn about our gender, 'race' and class positions as singular or discrete elements; they are inextricably bound together, each one being dependent on the others for definition and clarification. I mentioned earlier my role as a witch at school. This is of course both a gendered and a racialized term with its own long history of persecution and oppression in Western culture, and mythic status and celebration in some African cultures. Black women are brought up in a value-laden, cultural, social and political context in which masculine behaviours are defined as being distinct from feminine, and attributes of Blackness are distinguished from 'whiteness': in each of these pairings, 'woman' and 'Black' are subordinated and denigrated even whilst being fetishized and desired.

The privileging of gender in a hierarchy of oppression where the primacy of ' race', gender and class are perceived as being in contestation has been a contributory factor in the stifling of 'white' feminist discussions of 'race'. Although the foregrounding of gender and sexuality in 'white' feminist discourse may be attributed to the predominance of psychoanalytic theory as a framework within which to examine women's oppression, such an exclusionary emphasis is unwarranted inasmuch as the ideological systems and the psychic mechanisms which produce and reproduce 'Blackness' and 'whiteness' are implicated in Freud's use of, and 'white' feminists' avoidance of, detailed analysis of the trope of 'the dark continent'.[3] I shall discuss this point in more detail later since the question of who or what constitutes the 'dark continent' is crucial to this study of the textual annihilation of Black women on film.

While Jane Gaines remains sceptical about the use of psychoanalytic theory in analysing 'race', feminism and film, African-American feminists Hortense Spillers and bell hooks have both poblematized psychoanalysis and its potential usage in Black cultural criticism. Although this debate seems to have mainly taken place in relation to the examination of Black people's literary works, the comments point to wider critical concerns. Bell hooks advocates the strategy of consistently challenging the notion that all major thought-systems originated with Europeans, and she maintains that the idea of 'white' people – predominantly, but not exclusively men – as Authors and Initiators characterizes notions of 'white' intellectual superiority and is embedded in academic discourse:

> we don't have to see white people as inventing psychoanalysis . . . we have to disrupt the whole discourse on psychoanalysis by saying that in fact racism determines the fact that we see psychoanalysis as white, as something not coming from people of colour.
>
> (Childers and hooks 1990: 66)

Hortense Spillers poses the problem in different terms:

> Is the Freudian landscape an applicable text (to say nothing of appropriate) to social and historic situations that do not replicate moments of its own origins and involvements?
> (1990: 129)

and then proceeds to reassess radically what psychoanalytic theory can offer to the understanding of 'race', class and gender relations historically. Spillers points to the way in which the Oedipal moment was radically disrupted for Africans who experienced European slavery. The Oedipus complex is fundamental to the psychoanalytic explanation of the entry of the infant into adult subjectivity. Spillers highlights the contradictions between the social and symbolic realms within the culture of slavery, in which Black women had no maternal rights and the Name of the Father established property rights through ownership of human commodities. She contends that since slavery precluded the African-American male from participating in the social fabrications of the Name of the Father and the Law of the Father, slave children (and their heirs) have a different relation to the patriarchal symbolic realm, the pre-existing social order. In this set of relations, femininity and masculinity were constructed through the experience of a double paternity: that is the African father's *banished* presence and name, and the counterfeit European father/master's contemptuous presence. In many 'white'-authored texts in which Black people appear, the Oedipal triad is rarely achieved since the Black father is either non-existent (un-named) or banished from the scene, and Black characters such as those Whoopi Goldberg plays have no families or even surrogate families from Black communities.

Outside the frame of feminism, racism, fantasy and representation have been tackled within a psychoanalytic framework by both Black and 'white' writers. Besides Spillers and hooks cited above, other important studies in the psychoanalysis of racism are Joel Kovel's book on 'white' racism (1988), which attempts a Marxist/psychoanalytic interrogation of 'white' racist ideologies, and Sander Gilman's essays on the representation of Black women in nineteenth-century European culture, centring on the concept of projection and fantasy (1985). Of Black writers to use psychoanalysis to examine racism, one of the most notable has been Frantz Fanon.

Fanon's work refers to his analytic practice and how this contributed to his understanding of anti-colonial politics. In his Lacanian-inspired psychoanalytic account of the relationship between the Black male body and the threat it poses to 'white' male subjectivity, Fanon clearly identifies Black men as being the 'white' man's Other. In a lengthy footnote discussing the mirror phase, Fanon notes how the Black man is seen purely in terms of his corporeality: '. . . for the white man The Other is perceived on the level of the body image, absolutely as the not-self – that is, the unidentifiable, the unassimiable.' (1986: 161) In this context, the significance of the mirror phase is that it provides an illusory coherent identity for 'white' male identity. Drawing on the analogy between the mirror phase and the illusion of wholeness that is provided through narcissistic identification in the cinema, it would seem logical that anything which disturbs that deluded sense of order would be subject to denial.

About Black women, Fanon assures us, he knows little. Although his work is not without its problems, particularly for feminists, Fanon is very clear about how sexuality is implicated in racism (Fanon 1986, especially Ch. 3).

Noting the difficulties involved, and not wishing to dismiss an entire body of work for its ethnocentrism (or its phallocentrism for that matter), I would refer back to Cornel West's comments about the necessity for racially recasting the terms, and attempt to expose the substructure of certain fundamental critical paradigms.

Although originally published in 1974, and despite continual revisions and critiques since then, Laura Mulvey's essay 'Visual pleasure and narrative cinema' remains a significant reference-point for feminist film criticism. This influential essay noted the representation of the heterosexualized female body as an essential component of most mainstream cinema, a re-presentation for male consumption. Mulvey described and analysed the gendering of the 'Look' but did not suggest how this might be racially differentiated.

Drawing on Freud's theory of infantile sexuality, Mulvey sought to explain the pleasure gained from looking at films in the cinema. Freud posited that the pleasure of looking – referred to as scopophilia – is a fundamental component of our sexual disposition, and that it is related to the child's desire to observe the primal scene. Mulvey related scopophilia to the process of watching films by suggesting a link between the self-contained private world as played out in front of us on the cinema screen, and the pleasure and desire invoked by the forbidden looking carried out as infants.

She noted that men are the major protagonists in most mainstream films and it is through the man's motivations, actions and thoughts that sense is made of the narrative: most often, the woman is there to stimulate the man into taking action. Fear, anxiety and desire are activated by the appearance of the female body and it is these psychic drives which propel the male character towards action stimulated by desire or aggression.

Mulvey postulated that the male unconscious has two possible escape routes from the anxiety stimulated by the woman's 'lack' of a penis. One route is continually to investigate Woman in an attempt to demystify her: in most mainstream films it is the female who is subjected to and subordinated by the male 'Look'. The woman is scrutinized by the male's Look as he attempts to assert control and to punish her for evoking and provoking (forbidden) desire.

It is also suggested that the male may avoid the anxiety of potential castration through fetishistic scopophilia which results in an over-valuation of the female image and is manifested in the cult of the female star – whose physical beauty becomes a source of satisfaction in itself. The male may set up the woman as a fetish, as a substitute for the penis she 'lacks', and which is the anatomical and symbolic sign of sexual difference. In these terms then, women's sexuality represents a threat, and a way of countering this threat is to locate the woman within the confines of the containing patriarchal structure of the monogamous heterosexual couple or family.

At this point it is necessary to stop and consider where women of African descent are positioned in this scenario. Leaving aside the question of spectatorship, I want to examine in more detail this question of the controlling 'white' male gaze in relation to Black women.

The first strategy of the male unconscious to which Mulvey refers – that of investigating the woman – is familiar in terms of the external reality outside of the world of film, since it is characteristic of nineteenth-century medical/scientific discourse, where the anatomical structure of Black women's genitalia was under constant scrutiny, publicly as well as in the laboratory (see Gilman 1985, Ch. 3).

Whereas 'white' women may be punished for the desire they provoke by death or disfigurement or by being abandoned, Black women are most frequently 'punished' by their symbolic annihilation and by their characters' peripheral status. In the past – particularly in North American cinema – as coons, servants and mammies, Black women were socially marginalized accessories to the dramas and intrigues of 'white' people's lives, the textual strategy being to downplay their existence as sexual beings. It is still 'white' middle-class men who have privileged access to looking rights and Black women who are most usually 'punished' for their instigation of complex anxieties and desires, by their continued marginalization and structured absence from films.[4]

As regards the second proposition, that of the valorization of the beauty of the female body, this is a position that is not available to African women to anything like the same extent that it is to European women. Talk of 'physical beauty' has to be problematized straightaway: the notion of feminine beauty has always been an oppressive concept for Black women in a European context. It has also, of course, been oppressive for 'white' women: but however hard a Black woman may try, she has always 'lacked' the essential prerequisite for European ideals of beauty, that is white skin. Historically, women of African descent have never been subject to 'overvaluation' in the same sense that 'white' women have, and comparatively few may be described as being part of 'the cult of the female star'.

Images of European women as the standard of beauty and desirability are pervasive, and few 'white' women seem to be aware of the ways in which they are imaged as the polar opposite of – yet dependent on – conceptions of Black women's sexuality and femininity. The role of Black women in providing a contrast for 'white' femininity is evidenced in Freud's work, where it is possible to detect notions of 'white' female sexuality – particularly that of the 'lower' classes – being conflated with the unknowable and fathomless sexuality of the 'primitive': this is made clear by the use of that colonial trope.

Freud posits that sexual control is contingent on a 'civilized' social structure, whereas sexual freedom is equated with the more 'primitive' peoples of Africa who are regarded as atavistic. Thus excessive (or at least less rigorously controlled) sexual activity is mapped onto the 'dark continent'.[5] The sexuality of the children in 'primitive' societies seems, Freud notes, 'to be given free rein', and although such freedom results in a society without neuroses, Freud speculates that this advantage may 'involve an extraordinary loss of the aptitude for cultural achievements' (Freud 1986b: 318). Fanon reiterates and elaborates on Freud when he states

> Every intellectual gain requires a loss in sexual potential. The civilized white man retains an irrational longing for unusual areas of sexual license, of orgiastic scenes, of unpunished rapes, of unrepressed incest. . . . Projecting his own desires onto the Negro, the white man behaves 'as if' the Negro really had them.
>
> (Fanon 1986: 176)

Freud's 'dark continent', though, was consciously referring to 'white', European women, and their involvement in the literal and figurative annihilation of Black women needs to be interrogated. In terms of representation, Black and 'white' women are linked by their common unknowability, their instigation of castration anxiety and provocative sexuality: this link is predicated on an oppositional relation rather than a relation of complementariness.

For 'white' men, 'white' women are both Self and Other: they have a floating status. They can re-enforce a sense of self through a common racial identity, or threaten/disturb that sense through their sexual otherness. Additionally, when a 'white' woman indulges in behaviour which may be seen as problematizing controlled and controlling racially determined heterosexual relationships, she may be held responsible for potentially reversing the progress of 'white' supremacy. By behaving 'badly' – for example, by being sexually attracted by a Black man, or by being a prostitute or lesbian – the 'white' woman illuminates the precarious nature of 'white' people's claim to superiority since she is a reminder that things could slip back, regress to a 'primitive', 'dark' condition. For the 'white' male, the racial Otherness of Black-ness, the oppositional racial relation, interacts with the sexual difference of woman-ness and precipitates a crisis of misrecognition and disavowal.

The distinctions between competing types of 'white' femininity may be clarified through Blackness: this seems to account for a film like Jonathan Demme's *Something Wild* (1986), where a 'white' woman's sexuality is identified as wild and excessive, and is predicated on her codification as a Black woman (see further Bailey 1988). There would seem here to be partial acknowledgement of the fact of 'white' women's dependency on the oppositionality of Black women's sexuality for a definition of their own. Historically, images of Black women and womanhood were constructed in order to validate and valorize its opposite in 'white' femininity and womanhood. The sexual oppositions pure/debased and Madonna/whore are operated through 'white' notions of Black femininity. In the case of *Something Wild*, perhaps we are witnessing another kind of 'passing', a trope for female duplicity and racial anxiety about the slippage from 'white' to Black: the downward slide from 'white' as pure to Black as debased. Black is dirty, sex is dirty and the two combine in Black sexuality. In film, the desire to engage in 'dirty' or transgressive sexuality may be projected onto the racial/sexual Other, so that explicit violent sexuality may be embodied directly in a Black woman as in, for example, Tina Turner in *Mad Max Beyond the Thunderdome* (George Miller and George Ogilvie 1985); Grace Jones in the title role of *Vamp* (Richard Wenk 1986); Simone (Cathy Tyson) in *Mona Lisa* (Neil Jordan 1986) or indirectly through the use of Black cultural iconography in a film such as *Something Wild*.

Characterizations of Blackness in theatrical, literary and visual culture draw on a repertoire of anxieties which are projected on to the African Other; anxieties marked by distortion, ambivalence and contradiction. These anxieties erupt in the form of 'positive' and 'negative' images, and through the denigration and the fetishization of 'Blackness' and are underpinned by guilt and denial.

In a discussion of 'Whiteness as an absent centre', Claire Pajaczkowska (1992) has indicated that the 'emotional state produced by denial is one of blankness' (p. 201) and it is this blankness which helps to sustain 'white' male identity as normal and as 'undefined'. Indeed, to return to *Heart of Darkness*, the blank spaces identified on the map of the world are the 'white' man's own, projected onto the Other. The blankness at the centre of the denial of racism, colonialism and imperialism serves to obscure a set of contradictory actions and fantasies which are sometimes unconscious, and which are manifest in the created representations of the African Other: representations which are projections of the 'good' and 'bad' split-off parts of the 'white' ego.

Although historically, as previously stated, women of African descent have never been subject to 'overvaluation' by Europeans in the same sense that 'white' women have, we have been subjected to other forms of this symbolic act. The form of overvaluation which we have endured has originated not only from sexual anxieties – as in the case of 'white' women – but also from racial fears. The idealization of the Black subject rests on the valorization of particular qualities and characteristics associated with slavism, representing an earlier, longed-for stage in human development where people were in touch with their feelings and responded instinctively, untouched by the trappings and attendant neuroses of Western civilization. This relates directly to Freud's remarks about 'primitive' sexuality, and to Fanon's comments on the split between (Black) body and ('white') mind, between sex and intellect, mentioned earlier. This form of idealization is based on the desire of 'white' people to achieve what is seen to be an unattainable ego-ideal – to be spontaneous, to be able to act on instinct, to be sexually uninhibited, to be spiritual and so on. The repressed but desired characteristics and qualities of the ego-ideal merge with the object of that idealization, and result in the introjection of the idealized object – the attempted absorption of what are seen as 'Black' characteristics. In order to illustrate this in more detail, I will now consider the way in which a contemporary Black actor, Whoopi Goldberg, operates through – and sometimes against – these motifs in her most successful film appearance to date: *Ghost*.

WHOOPI GOLDBERG AND *GHOST*

> The Negro is in demand . . . but only if he is made palatable in some way. Unfortunately, the Negro knocks down the system and breaks the treaties. Will the white man rise in resistance? No, he will adjust to the situation.
>
> (Fanon 1986: 176)

Ghost is a story about how love survives death. The 'white' male protagonist, Sam (Patrick Swayze), is killed in order to prevent him revealing the fraud initiated by a colleague at the financial institution where they both work. His lover Molly (Demi Moore), devastated by his murder, is contacted by Oda Mae Brown (Whoopi Goldberg) at the instigation of Sam's ghost who cannot settle until his murderer is brought to justice. Oda Mae is a phoney psychic who subsequently discovers that she actually does have the ability to speak with the dead and reluctantly participates in the search for Sam's killer. This is, of course, successfully achieved, and Oda Mae and Molly witness Sam's ascension to heaven, guided by bright white 'angels'.

Generally in 'white'-authored films, Black people appear on-screen isolated from their culture, their families and their iconography – except in the form of parody. This parodic element seems to me to be present in Goldberg's work through the way in which her performance/characterization in *Ghost* is distinctively 'Black'.

Since, as Cornel West puts it, '... Black peoples' quest for validation and recognition occurred on the ideological, social and cultural terrains of other neo-Black peoples' (1992: 26) strategies of cultural resistance were developed which simultaneously incorporated and rearticulated European ideologies and African heritage. The key modes of resistance were the development of distinctive practices – linguistic innovation, hairstyles, ways of moving, and other expressions of physicality, stylish dressing, sustaining intra-community dialogue and so on – which reconstructed the 'alien social space' within which African Americans found themselves. It is on this cultural terrain that Goldberg fashions her *Ghost* performance, taking on those resistances and developing them. I experience an uneasiness about this which comes from a sense that those elements of Black cultural expressivity and resistance to which West refers are turned back on us. So that, with hair, for example (a prime site of ideological contestation within Black communities) visual and verbal references to Black women's hairstyles in the film indicate that they are imitative and derisory. As regards dress and style, Oda Mae Brown's clothes range from the androgynous to the inappropriately feminine, at that end of the scale being ostentatious rather than stylish. Her heeled shoes cause her to walk in an odd, arthritic and uncomfortable manner. Oda Mae's use of language is amusing rather than subversive or disruptive of the social order. Importantly, her potential as a medium is fake until its authenticity is revealed by Sam, the film's 'white' male protagonist. Intra-community dialogue is restricted to the realm of comedy, and based on a corrupt version of Black spirituality. So, in those significant areas of resistant, potentially rebellious, African-American behaviour and expression, the nature of Oda Mae

Brown – and of Black America – is diminished through mockery and humour.

Most mainstream cinema perpetuates the naturalness of both 'white' supremacy and Black people's outsider status in the dominant social order. As in nineteenth-century pseudo-science, the stigmata of class and 'race' are identified and re-created in representation. Blacks of low social and economic status are characterized by physical/anatomical signifiers of their cultural distinctiveness such as rolling eyes, wide grins, Black vernacular and body movements because they are poor: thus Blackness and poverty become interchangeable terms with a naturalized, inevitable coexistence. As Oda Mae visually demonstrates on her walk across town from the ghetto to the financial district, she is out of place, not only in terms of her sexuality and her 'race' but also in terms of her class. Her intruder status is signified through her clothing: the bright fuschia-pink jacket she wears contrasts with the sombre greys that the 'white' people wear and the discomfort caused by the heeled shoes and pencil skirt make her walk in a way which resembles that of a female impersonator, signalling an anxiety with the posture of femininity.

IMAG(IN)ING WHOOPI GOLDBERG

> It is scarcely possible to think of a black American actor who has not been misused: not one that has ever been seriously challenged to deliver the best that is in him. . . . What the black actor has managed to give are moments, created, miraculously, beyond the confines of the script; hints of reality, smuggled like contraband into a maudlin tale, and with enough force, if unleashed, to shatter the tale to fragments.
>
> (James Baldwin, quoted in Dyer 1986: 71)

Has Goldberg in some sense come to be seen as a Black archetype, representative of the essence of female Blackness itself?[6] In newspaper interviews, Goldberg is constructed as embodying 'Black' qualities, bearing a 'huge grin and popping eyes' (*You* magazine, *Mail on Sunday* 16 March 1986) her naturalness is emphasized time and time again as she denies any training or 'method' style preparation for her roles. The narrative of the poor Black who eventually made good is replete with examples of her earthiness, her triumph over deprivation caused by a drug habit, unemployment and teenage pregnancy. Her experience of motherhood at an early age and a broken marriage of course fits with the Black welfare mother stereotype. Although the fact that her daughter also got pregnant at a young age, repeating the cycle of Black deviancy from the patriarchal norm, emphasizes the inevitability of it all, at the same time Goldberg's experiences are narrativized so as to perpetuate the fantasy that her success is due to North American meritocratic society.

In the interviews held with Goldberg before and after the acclaim received for *Ghost* there are striking, indicative descriptions of her physical appearance: 'Plain as button . . . the face of a street urchin with a Topsy hairdo' (*Daily Express* 20 January 1986).

'Perhaps it is the kind of face only a mother can love. But it's lit with a smile as wide as a frying pan . . . braided locks tumble down her face like a liquorice fountain' and '. . . *she smiles so long and slow that you think her teeth will catch cold.*' (original italics) (*Daily Mirror* 19 September 1990). Frantz Fanon refers to how important it is for 'white' people to see Black people grinning. The African, without responsibilities, in a condition of primitive, blissful simplicity was said by 'whites' to be truly happy. This is the basis for those stereotypes of the happy, smiling, clown-like Black figure: and it is significant that the major Black female star is a comic performer rather than a serious dramatic actor.

'I prefer to see myself as sexless and colourless' says Whoopi Goldberg, according to a feature in *The Mail on Sunday* (16 March 1986). This statement may be regarded as naive or knowing or an ambivalent expression of both. The *Village Voice* (17 January 1989) seem not to view her as human in their caption of her photograph: 'from duckling to eagle'. The *Village Voice* reporter also notes that having played a number of spies and police officers, 'she gets shot at and beaten more than any woman I can think; she also defends herself and goes on the attack more' (ibid.). Apart from suggesting that the precarious nature of Black women's existence is mirrored in Goldberg's characters, who are often in danger of being annihilated, this indicates the masculinized roles in which Goldberg is cast. *Village Voice* reports that Goldberg does not care if she is thought of as androgynous: I would suggest that this androgyny is symptomatic of 'white' Hollywood's inability to deal with the implications of representing Black women on film. In this scenario, Goldberg may be seen as an embodiment of the way in which Black women are represented as alien to notions of femininity, womanhood and mothering such as are amplified and continually elaborated in representations of 'white' womanliness.

In the films *Fatal Beauty* (Tom Holland 1987), *Jumpin' Jack Flash* (Penny Marshall 1987), *The Telephone* (Rip Torn 1988) and *Ghost* (1987), Goldberg wears clothing which obscures and de-emphasizes her body shape. In *Jumpin' Jack Flash*, *Fatal Beauty* and *Ghost* we see her leave her regular loose, 'masculine' attire and assume the 'masquerade' of femininity. Thus masculinity and femininity become reduced to expendable, changeable signifiers. However, Goldberg's discarding of masculinity and her assumption of femininity result in inappropriate female behaviour, marking her out as an imposter and punishing her attempted assumption of the role of object of ('white') male desire. In *Jumpin' Jack Flash*, for example, her shimmering blue, tightly fitting dress is torn to pieces in a shredding machine. Her 'feminine' clothing in *Ghost* invites derision, the uncomfortable shoes forcing her to walk in a manner associated with a man in drag.

In these instances though, the *denial* of sexual difference is not liberating since this form of androgyny is predicated on a masculinizing of the feminine in order to diminish Black women's threat, which in this case is based on sexual and racial difference. As a desexualized but masculinized Black woman, Goldberg becomes a non-threatening stand-in for Black men – woman as a castrated man because Black male sexual and political potency must not be realized and has to be continually forestalled – as well a representational denial of Black women's sexuality/fertility. Androgyny can represent a destabilizing of absolutist categories of sexual difference but ends by re-enforcing them. Thus her non-sexuality is not liberating, merely obscuring – a screening device. She is a Black woman without Blackness and woman-ness: a contemporary echo of the asexual mammy, a refiguring of the double negation.

Demi Moore's gamine appearance gives Molly a boyish but vulnerable quality, which stands in stark contrast to Ode Mae's street-wise feisty Black woman. The vocal style, clothes and demeanour of the two women are diametrically opposed. This opposition – emphasized through racial difference – does not give rise to any dilemma for Sam, since there is no question of there being any sexual attraction between him and Oda Mae. The threat of sexual rivalry with Molly is diminished through various strategies: Goldberg's characterization of criminality, the absence of sexualized situations for Oda Mae and thus her sexual potential is disavowed. There is another aspect to the relationship between Molly and Oda Mae. Mary Anne Doane points to the manner in which Black women have in the past served as a:

> textual echo of the white female protagonists, or at least, an echo of what they have allegedly lost as the price of their middle-classness. The intuitive knowledge or maternal power credited to the black woman acts as a measure of the distance between the white bourgeois woman and the nature or intuition she *ought* to personify.
>
> (Doane 1991: 240)

The extraordinary scene in *Ghost* where Sam re-colonizes Black women through merging his body with that of Oda Mae Brown is inflected with the psychic processes of repression, projection and introjection. What seems to be happening is complex and contradictory and thus characterizes some of the ambivalence that exists in the matrix of relations between Black/White/women/men. Goldberg's Oda Mae Brown is the servant of the 'white' man and woman, the go-between who is used to get in touch with their emotional centre and help to connect with each other. Molly and Sam as two gendered sides of the split 'white' self are unable to communicate fully when Sam is alive: he cannot bring himself to utter 'I love you' but hides behind the Latinate 'ditto', and when he is dead, she cannot 'see' or 'hear' him. Even their initial lovemaking is figured through a clay phallus, to the sound of The Righteous Brothers.[7] This composite 'white' self can only fully articulate its emotions through the comic, disreputable but spiritually gifted medium Oda Mae Brown. Oda Mae is morally redeemed by Sam – she is not a fake, she does some good by donating money to the poor – even as she is the instrument of his humanization.

Having been morally reclaimed by the 'white' man, Oda Mae gives over her body to him so that he can make physical contact once more with his lover. The audience is allowed to see what Molly feels, so that although in terms of the text's internal reality, established within the narrative, Molly is really embracing Oda Mae, we see Molly embracing Sam. The textual disavowal of the potential sexual charge between Molly and Oda Mae in this scene is accomplished by seamless editing and imaginative dexterity. For the film to have allowed us to witness the ultimate sexual transgression – lesbian sex across racial lines – would have been too threatening, so instead we are left to ponder: who is Molly caressing? A dead 'white' man or a living Black woman?

I've watched for the subtleties of Goldberg's performance and I admire her interpretive skills as a comic actor. She has managed to retrieve some meaning from otherwise mediocre scripts such as those of *Burglar*, *Jumpin' Jack Flash*, *Fatal Beauty* and *The Telephone.* In *Ghost*, she visually disrupts the grey, dull 'white' world with which we are presented and which is so virtuous on the outside but so corrupt on the underside. The 'white' lead characters look as though they have been made on a conveyor belt which produces characters designed to be pleasing to look at and to listen to: decor, clothing and vocalization are self-consciously understated, anything raucous or earthy is figured through Black people or expunged. As we subsequently learn though, the world of the 'white' all-American yuppie enacted before us, and the friendship between the men of that world, is evidently insincere and fabricated. The people of that world certainly have no sense of their place as 'white' people beyond their assumption of superiority. They are incapable of being self-reflexive about their ethnicity since they are not conscious of it: they are therefore unable to interrogate the 'whiteness' of their world.

In thinking about Whoopi Goldberg, I am not suggesting that she as an individual should be denounced for playing the roles she does or saying the things she is quoted as saying. It is an oversimplification of the issues to accuse Black performers of 'selling out', just as it is to celebrate Black actors just for having got there. The tendency to censure Black performers for taking on demeaning roles is problematic since little is gained from such condemnation by way of analytical insight into the material circumstances which produce imbalances in power relations, or the performance skills of the actor who attempts to imbue otherwise mundane scenarios with some meaning.

THE LAST WORDS

The choice of a comic/fantasy context diffuses the potentially disruptive impact that the intrusion of a Black character in an occasionally non-subordinate role into the lives of a 'white' heterosexual couple might have had. What issues are being avoided here by shying away from a serious dramatic genre? As noted above, the image of contented, comic Black people remains an important one. If we relate this back to the issue of the natural state of Blackness, the normalized characteristics of Black people from eighteenth- and nineteenth-century slavery, to contemporary symbolic slavery, then it can be read as meaning that Black people can 'put up with' subordination and deprivation and still remain good-natured rather than rebellious. Again this serves as a comforting mechanism. The humour which emanates from the Black characters also encourages the notion that when Black people get together, they are an amusing spectacle – which is borne out by the characterizations of Oda Mae's two 'mammy' assistants.

It is crucial within textual analyses to examine the assumptions of 'white' supremacy as manifested in visual culture such as television and film as well as in literature and history. In carrying out such analyses, the objective is not just to expose that which was previously concealed, but also to recast the terms on which theoretical positions are constructed. Although much of what I have discussed in this chapter relates to the way in which issues of 'race' are marginalized in critical analysis, and I have not attempted to address the intersections of class and other facets of identity which fragment the category 'woman', I regard it as vital to work from within a framework which is able to recognize gender and class issues as interacting with ethnicity.

A cinematic text cannot be exclusively attributed to those directly involved in the production of the film but should be analysed as part of a complex web of inter-related experiences and ideas, fantasies and experimental expressions of desire, anxiety, fear and denial that need to be located in their historical, political and social contexts.

NOTES

A revised version of this chapter appears in *Fear of the Dark: Race, Gender and Sexuality in the Cinema* (Routledge, 1995).

1 The San were named 'Bushmen' by Europeans.
2 Whether there is any empirical evidence to support or deny such assertions is irrelevant: the fact that these notions are considered meaningful, are still perpetuated either directly or indirectly and are still the subject of many jokes, is the significant issue.
3 In her *Femmes Fatales: Feminism, Film Theory, Psychoanalysis* Mary Ann Doane (1991) devotes a whole chapter to a consideration of racial and sexual difference in the cinema, using the 'dark continent' as a starting point for her discussion.
4 Jane Gaines suggests that in analysing the 'Look', the psychoanalytic model may not be able to examine 'how some groups have historically had the licence to "look" openly while other groups have "looked" illicitly' (Gaines 1988: 24). The issue of the Black male look at 'white' females is still a significant uncharted area in film criticism.
5 It is interesting to note that Freud equates those of 'the lower strata of civilized races' with the 'races at a low level of civilization'. Sander Gilman demonstrates that much of nineteenth-century scientific thought linked the differentials of 'race', class and gender, in order to identify those deemed to be instrumental in bringing about social degeneracy. However, Freud, he claims, recognized that anthropological and scientific models of degeneracy were informed by political imperatives and that Freud saw 'the degenerate not as a real biological category but as a concept revealing of a specific understanding of the historical process' (Gilman 1985: 191ff).
6 Originally named Caryn Johnson, Whoopi Goldberg initially gained attention as a stage entertainer, becoming the first Black female stand-up comic since Moms Mabely whose career started in the 1930s. For more on Jackie 'Moms' Mabely, see Bogle (1980). There are further details on Whoopi Goldberg in Bogle's comprehensive book *Blacks in American Films and Television: An Illustrated Encyclopedia* (1988) and in his revised edition of *Toms, Coons, Mulattoes, Mammies and Bucks: An Interpretive History of Blacks in American Films* (1991).
7 The use of that music on the soundtrack is interesting since it is symptomatic of the 'white' music industry's predatory relationship with Black music. The Righteous Brothers, through their very name and the way in which they were marketed as a 'white' duo with a 'Black' vocal sound, mark out the boundaries for Black cultural expression. The 'authentic Black' sound is too raw, too difficult for the 'white' audience and has to be mediated by 'whiteness'. Thus desire and envy of Black cultural expression runs alongside the need to appropriate and control that experience. Here again we learn about Whiteness through its oppositional juxtaposition with Blackness.

BIBLIOGRAPHY

Bailey, C. (1988) 'Nigger/lover – the thin sheen of race in *Something Wild*', *Screen: the Last Special Issue on Race?* 29(4).

Beckles, H. (1989) *Natural Rebels: A Social History of Enslaved Black Women in Barbados*, London: Zed Books.

Bogle, D. (1980) *Brown Sugar: Eighty Years of America's Black Female Superstars*, New York: Da Capo Press.

Bogle, D. (1988) *Blacks in American Films and Television: An Illustrated Encyclopedia*, New York: Fireside.

Bogle, D. (1991) *Toms, Coons, Mulattoes, Mammies and Bucks: An Interpretive History of Blacks in American Films*, New York: The Continuum Publishing Company.

Brantlinger, P. (1987) 'Victorians and Africans: the genealogy of the myth of the dark continent' in H. L. Gates (ed.) *Race, Writing and Difference*, London: University of Chicago Press.

Childers, M. and hooks, b. (1990) 'A conversation about race and class' in M. Hirsch and E. Fox Keller (eds) *Conflicts in Feminism*, New York: Routledge.

Conrad, J. (1989) *Heart of Darkness*, London: Penguin.

Doane, M. A. (1991) *Femmes Fatales: Feminism, Film Theory, Psychoanalysis*, London: Routledge.

Dyer, R. (1986) *Heavenly Bodies*, New York: St. Martin's Press.

Ellison, R. (1964) *Shadow and Act*, New York: Random House.

Fanon, F. (1986) *Black Skin, White Masks*, London: Pluto Press.

Freud, S. (1986a) *Historical and Expository Works on Psychoanalysis* (trans. James Strachey) London: Penguin.

Freud, S. (1986b) 'The question of lay analysis: conversations with an impartial person' in A. Dickson (ed.) *Historical and Expository Works on Psychoanalysis* (trans. James Strachey) London: Penguin.

Fusco, C. (1988) 'Fantasies of oppositionality: reflections on recent conferences in Boston and New York', *Screen: the Last Special Issue on Race?* 29(4).

Gaines, J. (1988) 'White privilege and looking relations: race and gender in feminist film theory', *Screen: the Last Special Issue on Race?* 29(4).

Gilman, S. L. (1985) *Difference and Pathology: Stereotypes of Sexuality, Race and Madness*, New York: Cornell University Press.

Goldwater, R. (1987) *Primitivism and Modern Art*, Cambridge, MA: Belknap Press.

Gould, S. J. (1981) *The Mismeasure of Man*, New York: Norton.

Hill Collins, P. (1991) *Black Feminist Thought*, London: Routledge.

Kovel, J. (1988) *White Racism: A Psychohistory*, London: Free Association Press.

Mulvey, L. (1985) 'Visual pleasure and narrative cinema' in B. Nichols (ed.) *Movies and Methods*, Vol. II, Berkeley, CA: University of California Press.

Pajaczkowska, C. and Young, L. (1992) 'Racism, representation, psychoanalysis' in J. Donald and A. Rattansi (eds) *'Race', Culture and Difference*, London: Sage.

Spillers, H. J. (1990) ' "The permanent obliquity of an in(pha)llibly straight": in the time of the daughters and the fathers' in C. A. Wall (ed.) *Changing Our Own Words*, London: Routledge.

Ware, V. (1992) *Beyond the Pale: White Women, Racism and History*, London: Verso.
West, C. (1992) 'The new cultural politics of difference' in R. Ferguson (ed.) *Out There: Marginalization and Contemporary Cultures*, New York: MIT Press.

Index